Telephone Triage in an Ophthalmic A & E Department

Telephone Triage in an Ophthalmic A&E Department

Janet Marsden

Clinical Nurse Specialist, Manchester Royal Eye Hospital

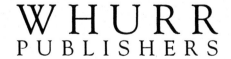

WHURR
PUBLISHERS

© 2000 Whurr Publishers Ltd
First published 2000 by
Whurr Publishers Ltd
19b Compton Terrace
London N1 2UN England, and 325 Chestnut Street, Philadelphia PA 19106, USA

Reprinted 2000 and 2002

British Library Cataloguing in Publication Data
A catalogue record for this book is available from the British Library.

ISBN 1 86156 151 2

Contents

Preface

In all accident and emergency (A&E) situations, staff need to be able to identify those patients whose needs are urgent and those who need less immediate attention. The almost universal strategy for achieving this is known as triage. The triage role has become an integral part of the nurses' role and contributes to the effective and timely care of patients presenting to the ophthalmic A&E service at Manchester Royal Eye Hospital.

The development of the researcher's department has led from a traditional walk-in service, staffed by doctors who examined and treated all patients, to the formation of a dual service. The Emergency Eye Centre, staffed by nurse practitioners who examine all patients and make decisions about treatment and referral, operates as a walk-in service for patients. The Acute Referral Centre (ARC) is run in conjunction with this, by a nurse practitioner and support staff along with medical staff, accepting patients referred by health professionals such as general practitioners (GPs), optometrists and nurse practitioners by telephone.

The formalization of this system of telephone advice in one area of the service led to the formalization of this previously unrecognized role in the Emergency Eye Centre. Telephone triage within the A&E service consists of eliciting information by questioning the patient or health-care professional about the perceived problem and making decisions on the most appropriate form of management. The patient is advised whether to attend the department or one geographically nearer to him or her, whether to consult their GP or whether to wait for the problem to resolve. Health-care professionals are advised whether the referral is appropriate for the service, and if not, how and where to refer appropriately. Advice may be given and treatment options suggested in order to obviate the need for an appointment; alternatively an appointment may be given.

Formalized telephone triage is a fairly new concept in the A&E service, even though it has been an informal strategy, here as in other areas of practice, for many years. Although the nurses within the service feel that they are able to elicit the information needed to make accurate and safe telephone triage decisions, there has been no investigation of this. It is clear that practitioners within the ophthalmic A&E service need to be very sure that patients who are at risk of losing their vision, or who have a problem that needs treating urgently, are identified – good questioning skills and a great deal of experience are needed. There appears to be little research available that investigates the accuracy of telephone triage decisions in any area of nursing practice.

This study, therefore, investigates the telephone triage decisions of nurse practitioners in the ophthalmic A&E service. A secondary analysis of data from one month was undertaken to reveal the range of diagnostic presentations to the departments (the ARC and the EEC). An analysis of the telephone triage sheets and correlation with the eventual diagnosis recorded for patients attending the A&E service was used to investigate referral patterns to the service and the accuracy and safety of the telephone triage decisions. Interviews were undertaken with the nurse practitioners to examine the process of telephone triage decision-making and some of their perceptions of the telephone triage procedure.

The study concludes that patients present to the A&E service with a vast range of ophthalmic problems, ranging from very minor conditions to sight-threatening emergencies. Decisions made at telephone triage appear to be both safe and accurate, and the provisional diagnosis or idea of the patient's problem arrived at by the nurse practitioner reflects the eventual diagnosis in a high proportion of cases. It appears that nurse practitioners have problems in obtaining an accurate history on which to base a telephone triage decision in some cases, this being particularly notable in some cases where the referrer is a GP. Some theories about expert knowledge and decision-making are propounded by other writers. The nurse practitioners use a process of hypothesis testing, a systematic and complex framework for decision-making, and demonstrate a reflective process of knowing.

The study informs and reassures practitioners, managers and users of the service of the validity and safety of telephone triage when undertaken by expert nurses in this area, and reinforces the literature surrounding expert nurse decision-making in practice.

There is little literature about the accuracy and safety of telephone triage decisions, and research in other areas of nursing practice is urgently needed in order effectively to validate this growing strategy.

Chapter 1

Personal location and literature review

Personal location

It is often perceived that a proportion of patients who attend Manchester Royal Eye Hospital's accident and emergency (A&E) service attend inappropriately, for problems that might be treated by their General Practitioner (GP). The patient's registration with a GP, while putting the GP under an obligation to that patient, does not, however, put the patient under an obligation to the GP; thus many attend the service for a second opinion (Jones & McGowan 1989). In ophthalmology, many people attend A&E because they are aware of the reputation of the Eye Hospital and feel that they will receive better care than from their GP. The perception of Green and Dale (1990) and many others, of the patient as an inappropriate attender, is not shared by the patient, so it can be considered that he or she deserves the same care as those whose attendance is seen as being more appropriate.

As in most A&E departments, staff need to be able to identify those patients whose needs are urgent and those who need less immediate attention. The almost universal strategy for achieving this is known as triage. The triage system of prioritization was formalized in the researcher's department in 1986. All patients had previously been assessed by an experienced nurse with a specialist qualification in ophthalmic nursing, and an informal system of triage was in place. The formalization enabled a better communication of the triage decision and the reasons for it, as well as ensuring continuity of care. The triage role has become an integral part of the nurses' role and contributes to the effective and timely care of patients presenting to the department.

The development of the researcher's department has led from a traditional 'walk-in' service, staffed by doctors who examined and treated all the patients, to the formation of a dual service. The Emergency Eye Centre is staffed by nurse practitioners, who examine all patients and make decisions about treatment and referral, assisted by support nurses, and operates as a walk-in service for patients. The Acute Referral Centre (ARC) is run in conjunction with this, by a nurse practitioner and support staff along with medical staff; it accepts patients referred by health professionals such as GPs, optometrists and nurse practitioners. Health professionals are expected to refer the patient by telephone to a nurse practitioner, who advises on the suitability and timing of the referral after eliciting various items of information.

The formalization of this system of telephone advice in one area of the service led to the awareness that giving advice by telephone to both patients and health professionals had always, informally, been a significant part of the nurse's role in the ophthalmic A&E department, but one which had not previously been acknowledged. Consequently, no formal recording of advice had been undertaken. Nurses in the Emergency Eye Centre discussed the formalization of this role and started to record details of telephone calls and of advice given. This strategy of formal telephone advice has been identified as an expansion of the triage role in other settings, most notably in general A&E departments, and has been designated 'telephone triage'.

In the researcher's department, telephone triage consists of eliciting information by questioning the patient or health-care professional about the perceived problem and making decisions on the most appropriate form of management. The patient is advised whether to attend the department or another geographically nearer to him or her, to visit the GP or to wait for the problem to resolve itself on its own. Health-care professionals are advised whether the referral is appropriate for the service and, if not, how and where to refer appropriately. Advice may be given and treatment options suggested in order to obviate the need for an appointment, or an appointment may be given.

It is clear that practitioners within the ophthalmic A&E service need to be very sure that patients who are at risk of losing their vision or have a problem that needs treating urgently are identified, so good questioning skills and a great deal of experience are needed.

Nurses in the researcher's department feel that they are able to elicit the information needed to make effective decisions about the most appropriate advice to give to the patient or the referring health professional. Unfortunately, there is no evidence to back up this contention, and the researcher feels that this is an area of practice demanding investigation. We, as practitioners, need to be assured that the advice we give and the decisions made about care are both appropriate and safe, so that sight-threatening conditions are appropriately dealt with. Managers and users of the service need to have the same information in order to assure a high level of confidence both in the service and in the advice given.

The perception of the need for more investigation in this area led to the formulation of three research aims:

1. to examine what conditions and problems present to the department (whether by telephone triage or by the patient presenting in person);
2. to examine the accuracy of the tentative diagnosis made by practitioners after the telephone conversation;
3. to examine the accuracy of the decision made to accept the patient for urgent treatment as opposed to suggesting strategies for less urgent referral.

A further aim was identified following a consideration of the literature relating to intuition and tacit knowledge within practice:

4. to explore the decision-making process adopted by nurses giving advice in telephone triage situations.

Literature review

The issue of appropriate attendance is a perennial problem for A&E departments, given the need to respond rapidly to cases that need such a response, and acceptably to those which are not in need of such emergency treatment. This review intends to examine the literature surrounding triage, a strategy that has proved to be an effective tool, both in the prioritization and targeting of care, and in the enhancement of patient satisfaction while in the department. 'Telephone triage' has developed following the success of triage and is becoming a recognized part of the role of the nurse in many specialist areas of practice. Decision-making is obviously crucial to both these processes and is made more difficult in telephone triage by the physical distance between nurse and patient. This literature review will therefore go on to discuss telephone triage, the decision-making processes involved in giving telephone advice, and decision-making in nursing in a wider context.

The workload of an A&E department is notable mainly by its variability: both the number of patients and their presenting problems vary considerably, and medical problems may range from the life threatening, taking large amounts of time and resources, to:

> seeming trivialities that should ostensibly have been treated by self-medication or sensible advice. (Read et al 1992)

In an attempt to dissuade patients with minor health problems from diverting medical attention from those with more serious problems, casualty departments were renamed accident and emergency departments following the publication of the Platt report in 1962 (Platt 1962). Attendance figures have risen continually since then (Milner et al 1988), and a number of studies have estimated that the proportion of attenders who could have been treated by their GP might be anything from 14% (Worth & Hurst 1989) to 68% (Cliff & Wood 1986). Wood and Cliff (1986) felt that A&E departments needed to find an urgent solution to the problem of providing services for patients with minor injuries who did not require hospital treatment.

The problem of rising numbers of what are perceived to be inappropriate attenders, plus a lack of resources, has led to overcrowding, long waiting times, frustration, aggression and stress, and the possibility that:

> in such conditions it is even possible that staff may fail to recognise, in their haste and harassment, that a patient is seriously injured or ill, and such a patient may die or suffer serious harm while in the waiting room. (Read et al 1992)

This has led to nurses in particular looking at possible solutions. One strategy that has gained wide acceptance, first in the USA and now in the UK, is the introduction of a triage, or prioritization, system for patients entering the department.

Historically, triage was used to describe the selection and grading of coffee beans (Thayre 1985). Military surgeons first used a triage system to decide on priorities of care in war situations, initially in the Napoleonic Wars and then to a much greater extent in World War I. Triage in this case was concerned with the rapid return of casualties to the battlefield, those who were least injured therefore being treated first, those who were salvageable with more intervention next, and those who needed major intervention being left until last. The more usually accepted version of triage was developed during the war in Vietnam. Patients were triaged into first, second and third categories and transported accordingly. Effective triage was generally credited with ensuring a relatively high level of medical care.

Various rationales and definitions of triage exist. Vayer et al (1986), examining triage from a military point of view, feel that the general theory of triage has remained constant:

> to allocate scarce resources in a manner which will provide the greatest good for the most people with minimum consumption of those resources.

From an A&E point of view, George (1976) felt that:

> triage is a process by which a patient is assessed on arrival to determine the urgency of the problem, and to designate appropriate health care resources to care for the identified problem.

Triage systems in the A&E department developed first in the USA following the Vietnam experience. Rund and Rausch (1981) and Thompson and Davies (1982) published books that were dedicated to the topic of triage and suggested various functions that formed part of the triage activity, including the early assessment of patient condition to determine the urgency of need for care, the control of patient flow through A&E, the application of first aid and the early initiation of diagnostic measures. They also felt that good public relations could be achieved by the obvious demonstration of concern, with consequent increases in patient satisfaction and opportunities for health education. Generally speaking, studies of triage undertaken in America agreed that nurse triage was safe and effective (Mills et al 1976, Rausch & Rund 1981).

Triage and literature about triage as an A&E strategy started to develop in Britain in the early 1980s. Blythin (1983) and Thayre (1985) both promoted triage as a strategy for the assessment of patients in the A&E department, identifying the same benefits as in the USA experience. In 1984, the Royal College of Nursing recognized three hospitals as practising nurse triage, and, on the whole, triage in the UK has been a nursing innovation.

Inappropriate attenders are obviously seen as a major problem in A&E departments, and some writers have examined triage as a tool for denying these patients care in the A&E department. Yates (1987) felt that (when identifying strategies to cope with high patient workload):

> only in the area of nursing service is there general
> disagreement as to the way ahead.

Yates believed that many nurses were happy with the traditional role of the nurse working for the doctor, and might be unhappy about the triage role (a situation in contrast to both nursing literature at the time and the development of this role in many areas). His promotion of triage roles appeared to be on the basis that the nurse might:

> indicate to the patient that their attendance in the A/E
> department is inappropriate and that management by a
> general practitioner would be advisable.

Yates surveyed 230 A&E departments to examine the view of medical staff with respect to the redirection of patients, reporting that 9% allowed nurses to refuse access to A&E and 41% would like to do so. Nurses were not surveyed about their views on this scenario.

Rock and Pledge (1991) identified that one of the activities of the triage nurse should be the redirection of inappropriate attenders without reference to a doctor and felt that:

redirection of inappropriate attenders to GP practices is
also beneficial in cutting down waiting times.

Most other literature is, however, concerned with quality of care and
patient satisfaction issues. Nurses, while recognizing that patients
attend A&E inappropriately, have looked at triage as a quality tool to
enhance care and satisfaction. Blythin (1983) looked at the usual
method of patient registration – reporting to a receptionist – and felt
that:

This unenviable method of registration, so typical of
many British A&E departments is tantamount to
providing the public with a second rate service.

Eaves (1987) was very concerned with the care of the 'inappropriate'
attender, stating that:

The common epithets of 'trivia' or 'rubbish' or even the
more respectable adjective 'minor' suggests that patients
given such labels receive a less than adequate service.

Nuttall (1986) wrote that:

triage has been advocated as an effective system for
reducing waiting times and ensuring that patients
presenting to emergency departments receive treatment at the appropriate time by appropriate personnel.

Blythin (1988) agreed with this, believing also that triage is useful
in stopping the possibly reduced care of patients with minor
problems:

triage seeks to challenge many of these problems by
establishing a system of patient management more
clinically sound and far more reliable than traditional
methods of patient reception.

He suggested that:

> it creates an environment which is conducive to high
> standards of care and management

and wrote that:

> at the very least, their condition has been noted and
> assessed by a person who is qualified to make such a
> judgement.

Jones (1986) proposed that a triage nurse in A&E could reduce waiting times by active intervention and the interpretation of investigations, leading to increased satisfaction for both patient and nurse. Bailey et al (1987) undertook a small-scale study of about 400 patients, timed their progress through an A&E department and looked at patient satisfaction using questionnaires. They found that the patients' time in A&E was reduced by 24% and that satisfaction with care increased. Mallett and Woolwich's study, published in 1990, also investigated the effect of triage on waiting time, discovering that the time the attender spent waiting to be clinically assessed by a health-care professional was shorter following the implementation of triage, although in 1986 the waiting time was the time taken to see a doctor, and in 1988 it was the time before seeing a triage nurse. Although the initial assessment in 1988 was not the actual consultation, as in 1986, this is still a clinical assessment, and priorities might be set and medical care initiated at that point.

The literature surrounding triage in A&E also emphasizes the accountability of nurses (Williams 1992) and the training and expertise needed by nursing staff in order to carry out the role effectively. Blythin (1988) suggests that the whole assessment process must incorporate a wide range of activities related to nurse–patient interaction, and believes that assessing patients in A&E is not a new concept to nurses, but an integral part of their role, which needs to be formalized using an evaluation of measurable and observable details combined with the subjective evaluation of an experienced nurse's response to a situation.

Triage is now widely accepted as a useful tool in the management of A&E departments, the issues of quality of care and patient satisfaction being more important than the redirection of patients in order to reduce waiting times. The Audit Commission report of 1992 states that triage is essential to quality of care, minimizing the risk of surprises in waiting areas and providing better communication and possibly better job satisfaction for nurses (Murphie & Marsden 1992).

The triage system has continued to develop over time to reflect particular settings and situations, different triage categories (1–3, 1–5, immediate/urgent/non-urgent and so on) being used in different areas, reflecting differing philosophies and workloads. A major expansion of the triage process has been the recognition and development of 'telephone triage'. As with mainstream triage, this development began in the USA, particularly in the A&E setting, although it is also recognized in other specialities such as primary care. Sweden has integrated telephone triage into its health-care system in such a way that:

> the receptionist nurse is the first practitioner in the Swedish health care system that a patient with a health problem is supposed to contact, normally through a telephone call. (Timpka & Arborelius 1990)

Timpka and Arborelius (1990) quote Marklund and Bengtsson (1989), who state that 20 million calls each year to health centres by a population of 8 million people are dealt with by receptionist nurses.

Telephone triage was first identified as a useful tool in the A&E setting in the UK by Buckles and Carew-McColl in 1991. Although giving advice by telephone has been an integral part of the nurse's role, it has not been one which is recognized as having a particularly distinct identity. Kernohan et al (1992) suggested that telephone advice is a part of the hidden workload of every speciality.

Glasper and McGrath (1993) state that:

> telephone triage involves health care professionals such as nurses, making decisions on the basis of a verbal history and giving appropriate advice that can fall into three areas prompting the client to seek immediate medical advice, which may be contained with first aid measures; directing the client to health professional but with less degree of urgency; or empowering the client to self care without the necessity of consulting a health care professional in person.

It thus combines all the perceived benefits; both for patients in terms of advice on first aid and strategies for treatment, and for the department in terms of the redirection of patients to a more appropriate setting.

Triage or advice-giving by telephone has the potential to be a valuable tool in many settings. Some authors stress that being able to solve problems by telephone will reduce attendance at A&E departments as well as inappropriate attendance. Buckles and Carew-McColl reported a reduction of 2% attendance at A&E after 1 year of telephone triage, 5% of patients who telephoned being redirected to other agencies.

Other writers stress the benefits for quality of care and patient satisfaction:

> meaningful telephone triage is a vital component of problem diagnosis, particularly in the primary care setting. If performed correctly, a telephone encounter will save valuable time and give the provider the pertinent information needed before the patient is seen or treated. (Stetson 1986)

There are many potential benefits identified for an expanded telephone triage role. Kernohan et al, in 1992, identified that 50% of patient problems presented by telephone to their paediatric A&E department were solvable without attendance at the unit. Sixty-eight per cent of all calls were identified as being genuine A&E problems. It thus seems that the necessity for some 'appropriate' attendance might be negated by good telephone advice.

Marklund et al (1990) found, in an evaluation of Swedish primary health-care telephone advice, that 98% of patients followed the advice given by telephone, and 91% were happy with the advice given. (The majority of the discontentment arose because the patient was given self-care advice or an appointment date more than 1 week away.)

Telephone triage activity might also be cost-effective. A quality review of the 'Sick Kids Hotline' in Toronto identified that the cost per call was less than $10, compared with a cost per visit of $100 (Wilkins 1992, quoted by Glasper & McGrath 1993). Other identified benefits of telephone triage were the feeling that it might enhance the patient empowerment aspects of the Patient's Charter, and might be marketable as a competitive feature of a service package when a Trust was tendering for contracts from purchasing authorities.

Disadvantages and changes of telephone triage are also highlighted in the literature. Dunn (1985) proposed that:

> the best rule for responding to a telephone request for
> medical advice is to tell the caller to come to the hospital
> because you cannot dispense or treat over the phone.

Dunn feels that only in life-threatening situations can the nurse safely give advice, but that life-threatening situations are difficult to determine over the telephone. Ultimately, she suggests that if the nurse must give advice over the telephone, calls and advice should be documented effectively.

Although the patients in Marklund et al's (1990) study were happy with advice given, the nurses were, in 10% of cases, not happy with the advice that they gave, as they were constrained by a lack of doctor appointments and were not able to give appointments to all those patients who, they felt, needed one. The nurses referred two-thirds of these patients to other centres. In 4% of cases, decisions were made that agreed with the subject's wishes, but which the nurse did not consider adequate.

This study was the only piece of literature identified that looked at the effectiveness of telephone triage in a 'real' (rather than simulated) situation. When doctors evaluated the cases, all but three calls (out of 494) were considered to have been handled medically correctly (when a doctor appointment was available), and all but two were referred to the correct level of care.

Glasper and McGrath (1993) felt that telephone triage might lead to problems of dissatisfaction, anxiety and litigation. In the primary care setting, the patient's notes are likely to be available, whereas in A&E, the patient is unknown and the telephone call may interfere with other work.

Wheeler (1989) believed that there was a failure to recognize the need to formalize telephone triage into an extended role, and that a proactive approach was needed, rather than the current trial-and-error situation. Glasper (1993) proposed that telephone triage in A&E is often undertaken by any passing health-care professional who is likely to be interested. This view is reinforced in a small-scale study by Crouch (1992), who reported that:

> the assessment of the patient's condition is purely subjective and relies on careful questioning to elicit facts. ... the general public have difficulty in assessing trauma and illness. What may be an important symptom to qualified personnel can be dismissed by the patient as a coincidence, or insignificant.

Crouch found that, on the whole, questioning was poor, often being carried out by unqualified personnel, and decisions were made hastily without eliciting the full facts.

A further study by Kunkler and Mitchell (1994) investigated the telephone advice given by A&E departments by telephoning the departments and asking for advice from a doctor regarding an imaginary relative. The authors found that 75% of the departments gave appropriate advice, but that the other 25% gave advice that was inappropriate and could, in some cases, have been dangerous. Student nurses and receptionists were involved in giving advice, and three departments informed the caller that they did not give advice by telephone.

Glasper (1993) concluded his review of telephone triage with the opinion that:

> imparting nursing information over the telephone is analogous to nursing with your eyes closed and your hands tied behind your back.

He recommended that a recognized triage course with clear learning outcomes, along the lines of the one established in Toronto, be established in the UK. A further recommendation is the design and use of adequate documentation for this role so that telephone triage can develop as it should. This echoes the recommendations of Knowles and Cummins (1984) in America, who addressed the same problems and recommended a designated telephone adviser, protocols for informed advice for common problems, and adequate documentation.

While some authors have examined the outcomes of telephone triage in terms of the benefits to the department and to the patient, others, perhaps recognizing the difficulties inherent in giving advice by telephone, as described by Glasper (1993), have examined the process of decision-making by nurses in this situation.

Timpka and Arborelius (1990) investigated decision-making in the primary care setting in Sweden and reported that telephone consultations were informing rather than counselling. Nurses described difficulties in drawing conclusions from, rather than gathering, data. Communication problems occurred, as did diagnostic dilemmas associated with not being able to see the patient. An uncomplicated decision strategy was apparent, and de Graafe (1989) suggests that this may be the result of nurses considering medical problems at a less complex level than doctors. Timpka and Arborelius (1990) found that dilemmas in decisions appeared to be caused by situational factors such as the availability of GPs, and suggested that an increase in medical responsibility should be accompanied by support measures such as training, as well as by day-to-day support.

Brennan (1992) examined the nursing process in telephone advice, reporting that although the nursing process illustrates the problem-solving aspects of nurses' work, intuitive aspects, experience and logic are ignored as a basis for practice. She suggests that experienced nurses have evolved beyond the use of the nursing process as a model, which is not helpful as a basis for assisting decision-making, and:

> need an elaboration of the nursing process model to provide articulation about their intuitive, quick grasp of situations and their ability to focus attention without unfruitful consideration of a large range of possible problem solutions.

Edwards (1994) undertook a study to:

> elicit the components of diagnostic reasoning utilised by experienced triage nurses when making triage dispositions via the telephone.

He felt that the nursing judgements involved are made in a crisis situation, in which accuracy and speed of assessment are needed, but are based on a minimum of information. Edwards found that:

> although deprived of the opportunity for methodolog-
> ical deliberation, nurses considered a broad and consis-
> tent range of components when making triage
> dispositions and that they did so within a systematic and
> identifiable framework.

Nurses generated hypotheses, using both the information given and single symptoms that the nurse perceived as being characteristic of a diagnosis. The probabilities of these hypotheses were weighed against the nurses' knowledge and experience. General information was gathered to 'buy time', and patient distress was considered, attending to verbal and non-verbal cues. Contextual factors such as those relating to 'chart characteristics, symptoms presentation and the possibilities offered by local health care facilities' were used to decide on the advice given, and much of the decision-making was based on experience. The ethical and emotional cost of decision-making was also highlighted.

Edwards' study involved only a small sample (10), and as the subjects were aware of the trial and simulation, the results might have been biased by this. In a simulation, any emotional response to the client and the effect of organizational factors are missing. However, Edwards suggests that further research is necessary to investigate the decision-making process involved in telephone triage in order more precisely to ascertain why particular decisions are made.

A large number of other authors have examined the knowledge and decision-making processes of nurses and others in more general terms. Polanyi (1967) identified a type of knowledge that he named 'tacit knowledge', defining it as that occurring when something is known only by relying on our awareness of it for attending to a secondary activity (proximal and distal knowledge). The skilled practitioner is unable to describe the skills used, and unable to describe the presuppositions of the decision-making.

Benner (1983) felt that clinical knowledge develops as practical and theoretical knowledge is applied, refined and extended in practice situations, going on to argue (1984) that expert practitioners view situations holistically and draw on past, concrete experience, whereas the merely competent or proficient must use conscious problem-solving. Benner asserts that:

> perceptual awareness is central to good nursing judge-
> ment and that this begins with vague hunches and
> global assessments that initially bypass critical analysis.

Benner's ideas about intuition were further refined in 1985, echoing Polanyi (1967) and stating that:

> all knowledge is not explicit. We have embodied ways of
> knowing that show up in our skills, our perceptions, our
> sensory knowledge, our ways of organising the percep-
> tual field. These bodily perceptual skills, instead of being
> primitive and lower on the hierarchy, are essential to
> expert human problem solving which relies on recogni-
> tion of the whole. (quoted by Brykczynski 1989)

Kenny (1994) identifies two forms of intuitive thinking, which she calls cognitive and empathetic. She defines cognitive intuition as: 'knowing, without fully understanding' and suggests that:

> Cognitive intuitive experiences are initially low key, as
> the thinker quietly draws together the various threads of
> theory in order to understand.

Empathetic intuition is felt to be similar to McCormack's (1993) description of the basis of understandng that something is wrong.

Kenny feels that:

> This type of intuitive feeling often occurs within the
> context of a nursing situation, and feeling, rather than
> conscious thinking, seems to predominate. Nurses know
> that there is something wrong but cannot explain what
> it is.

Schön (1987) states that professional education neglects tacit knowledge and gives privileged status to systematic, scientific knowl-edge, which may be of only marginal relevance to practice. He suggests that the expert practitioner uses a reflective process of 'knowing' and demonstrates reflection-in-action, stating (1991) that this is not just the application of theory to practice, but also the concept of thinking and adding to that theory while the action is occuring.

Meerabeau (1992) suggests, citing Atkinson et al (1977), that:

> tacit knowledge may be a positive asset, and is in fact the hallmark of a profession; the concepts used are those of indeterminacy and technicality. Technicality refers to procedures that can be mastered and communicated in the form of rules whereas indeterminacy refers to a variety of tacit and private knowledge which cannot be made wholly explicit. Many aspects of a profession can therefore be taught only through experience and close association with expert practitioners.

Whereas Polanyi feels that tacit decision-making cannot be verbalized, other authors feel that it can, although they have differing views on the effects of verbalization on decision-making. Henry et al (1989) reported that the verbalization of the process of decision-making makes little difference to proficiency or efficiency scores. Benner (1984) thought that the expert's skill level might fall if asked to verbalize while performing the skill, while, in contrast, Corcoran and Narayan (1988), cited by Orme and Maggs (1993), argue that thinking aloud can aid decision-making.

Other authors lay less stress on tacit or intuitive knowledge. Elstein and Bordage (1979) looked at physicians who saw themselves as making intuitive judgements based on knowledge and experience. An analysis of the decisions revealed that they were not using intuition but a cognitive strategy, the hypothetico-deductive approach. The practitioner builds hypotheses and then gains further cues on whether to refute or confirm these until a conclusion is reached.

This is echoed in work by Tanner et al (1987), which examined diagnostic reasoning in nurses and concluded that expert nurses activated diagnostic hypotheses early in an encounter and used systematic information-gathering to rule in or rule out hypotheses. They found that the greater the knowledge and experience of the nurses, the better was the systematic data acquisition and the greater the accuracy of the diagnosis. The presence of one 'symptom', a pivotal finding bridging the problem to the extensive knowledge of the expert, was described first by Eddy and Clanton (1979)and subsequently by Tanner et al (1987) and Edwards (1994).

In his study of decision-making in telephone triage, Edwards found that a wide range of factors – both medical and contextual – were used in arriving at a judgement, ethical and emotional factors also being apparent. Garthe (1984) states that it is the recognition of the ethical, legal and social responsibilities of nurses to clients that makes nursing decision-making unique. Farrington (1993) suggests that although Benner values expertise:

> decision making by intuitive means and the application
> of expertise are not necessarily indicators of expert
> clinical practice in nursing

citing Kahneman and Tvesky (1990), who point out that 10 years of experience may be 10 years of continuous development or 1 year of the same experience repeated 10 times. Farrington believes that the adaptation of heuristics, a rapid form of cognitive reasoning that is used in conditions of uncertainty or of the unavailability or indeterminacy of important information (Kahneman & Tvesky 1973), would enable:

> inferences and predictions to be made from the
> sometime scanty and unreliable data available. Such use
> of heuristics as a rapid form of reasoning and cognitive
> processing would enable the development of shortcuts
> to reduce complex problem solving to more judgmental
> operations and more effective decision making.

Kahneman and Tvesky's adjustment and anchoring heuristic, which reflects a tendency to make estimates from an initial value or anchor point and adjust them in the light of new information and the simulation heuristic, involving the construction of hypotheses, bears a strong resemblance to the hypothetico-deductive reasoning already described.

Finally, Orme and Maggs (1993) brought together expert clinicians to discuss decision-making. The group saw that effective decision-making was an integral part of the clinical role and felt that risk-taking was often involved (this not having been identified by other writers in this area, although they have acknowledged professional accountability). The process of decision-making was constant across clinical areas, but the pace was different, even within the same area. These authors reported that:

> expert decision making is dependent on an in-depth knowledge and experience of research and care provision for the group of patients/clients with whom the practitioner is working.

They also said that the environment within which the practice takes place is important and affects the quality of decision-making. Peer support and the opportunity for reflection, permission to take risks and supportive management all make a positive contribution to effective decision-making.

Orme and Maggs also identified a clear philosophy of care as being a very important contribution to effective decision-making. The group endorsed the importance of intuition in decision-making but felt that it would be impossible to analyse or quantify what the intuitive process might be, as it would thereby become conscious and no longer intuitive. They stressed that:

> before intuition can be of value, there must be a pre existing knowledge base which fosters the appropriate and relevant interpretation of information.

It seems therefore that tacit knowledge and intuition are accepted by most authors as being an integral part of expert decision-making, along with a pre-existing knowledge base and experience of the area of practice. The main area of disagreement concerns whether intuitive knowledge can, in fact, be explored by verbalization or other strategies, or whether to attempt to do so would render it invalid.

The areas of literature explored in this review have examined the concept of triage from a historical perspective, its refinement into a tool for use in A&E and the development of a strategy known as telephone triage. The process of decision-making by nurses, both in the telephone triage situation and in a wider context, has been discussed. It is obvious that there is room for further research in all areas, particularly in the area of telephone triage. It has not been possible to identify a study actively considering the effectiveness of the decisions made utilizing this system in the A&E setting. This is the area that is intended to provide the material for further study along with a further examination of the process of decision-making in telephone triage as recommended by Edwards (1994) following his research in this area.

Chapter 2
Methodology

The perceived lack of knowledge about the accuracy of telephone triage decision-making in general, and the researcher's practice area in particular, has led to the formulation of three research aims:

1. to examine what conditions and problems present to the department (whether by telephone triage or by the patient presenting in person);
2. to examine the accuracy of the tentative diagnosis made by practitioners after the telephone conversation;
3. to examine the accuracy of the decision made to accept the patient for urgent treatment as opposed to suggesting strategies for less urgent referral.

A further aim was identified following a consideration of the literature relating to intuition and tacit knowledge within practice:

4. to explore the decision-making process adopted by nurses giving advice in telephone triage situations.

Data collection methods

Collecting data to explore the first aim of the research involved examining the records of both areas of the A&E service and collecting the diagnoses that were recorded for each patient over a period of 1 month. Where the record within the department was incomplete or unclear, case notes or casualty cards were traced and the diagnosis recorded.

Aims 2 and 3 involved a secondary analysis of the same set of telephone triage records. The same period of 1 month was utilized as for aim 1. Secondary data analysis was undertaken in conjunction with other department records in order to correlate the provisional diagnosis with the actual diagnosis (for aim 2), and further examine the records of those patients who were accepted when they might safely not have been, or to whom advice or information was given (for aim 3).

Small group or individual interviews were undertaken that explored the nurses' ideas about their decision-making processes in relation to telephone triage in order to gather information for aim 4.

Location

The location for the study was Manchester Royal Eye Hospital's A&E service. This service includes the Acute Referral Centre (ARC), which accepts referrals of patients with acute problems, solely by telephone, from health-care professionals – GPs, hospital doctors and optometrists as well as nurse practitioners. The telephone referral process is known as telephone triage as information elicited from the referrer enables the nurse practitioner to make decisions concerning what course of action to take for each particular patient. This may be to accept the patient for an appointment immediately or within 48 hours, or to give advice on treatment or referral to more appropriate areas of the service. The other part of the service is the Emergency Eye Centre, which is a walk-in, nurse practitioner-led department. Patients are assessed by nurse practitioners and decisions made about treatment or referral.

A significant amount of telephone triage is undertaken in this department, advising patients when and where to attend for treatment or alternative strategies such as advice or reassurance. A certain amount of contact with health-care professionals also takes place, particularly out of normal working hours (at evenings and weekends).

Target population

The target population for the study's first three aims are the subjects of telephone triage:

- in the ARC, mainly health-care professionals with a small number of self-referring patients;
- in the Emergency Eye Centre, mainly patients who are self-referring, with a small number of health-care professionals.

It was considered by the researcher that 1 month's telephone triage records would provide a convenience sample that was large enough to provide an overview of the service, but not too large to handle within the limited time and resources available. (This sample provided 303 records from the ARC and 158 from the Emergency Eye Centre.) The target population for aim 4 includes the nurse practitioners working within both areas – a total of six nurses.

Philosophical paradigm

In order to explore further the possibilities of research in this area, it is necessary to examine some of the many philosophical approaches to research, or paradigms, and attempt to identify which approach most reflects both the beliefs of the researcher and the aims and constraints of the area for research.

Guba (1990) suggests that the term 'paradigm', in its most generic sense, refers to:

> a basic set of beliefs that guides action, whether of the everyday garden variety or action taken in connection with a disciplined enquiry.

The traditional set of beliefs that have tended to underpin scientific enquiry are those now known as positivism. Positivism has a belief that a single reality exists, one driven by natural laws that can be discovered by scientists in order ultimately to control and predict the behaviour of the natural world. The scientist must obtain information without interacting with it in any way so that it remains 'pure' knowledge, and objectivity and the elimination of researcher bias are necessary. Empirical methods must be used to eliminate the possibilities of any bias in order to achieve this pure scientific knowledge. Collin (1985) states, in relation to social science research compared with 'pure' science research:

> positivism explicitly embraced the view that one and the
> same set of scientific methods must be used in the two
> fields. The secrets of human action should be unveiled
> with the same intellectual tools that had proved so
> powerful in natural science.

Phillips (1990) links the lessening in influence of positivism to developments in scientific knowledge after World War II. Science developed to the extent that theories were accepted about events that could not be observed to be true, such as those in the field of subatomic particle physics, and this led to the acceptance that the positivist view of research and knowledge was badly flawed. He suggests that science, both natural and behavioural, would have had trouble extending into new areas had this position continued to be accepted.

Other paradigms or philosophical approaches to research have emerged, and their introduction:

> undermines the tacit but widely held belief that there is
> only one dependable way to know, something vaguely
> called 'the scientific method'. (Eisner 1990)

Eisner goes on to suggest that a critical consciousness of a paradigm is not likely to occur if it has no competitors, and the emergence of other paradigms forces the examination and defence of the researcher's position and, therefore, better understanding.

Two of these paradigms or sets of beliefs are known as post-positivism and constructivism. Post-positivism may be thought of as a modified form of positivism which accepts that it is impossible for humans fully to understand the real world, and that one will never be sure that the ultimate truth has been found. It still suggests, however, the concept of a single reality. Post-positivism recognizes the impossibility of the researcher stepping outside the 'self' to become totally objective, and suggests that the ideal is to be as neutral as possible, while 'confessing' one's own position. It relies on the 'critical community' to maintain objectivity.

The constructivist position is based on the idea that facts are true only within some theoretical framework, and that there are always a number of theories that can explain a series of facts. This means that no unequivocal answer is ever possible and:

> 'Reality' can be 'seen' only through a window of theory,
> whether implicit or explicit. (Guba 1990)

This leads to the suggestion that reality can also only be seen through a window of values, and that the research is likely to be shaped by the interaction between the researcher and the subject, thus making any findings not what is actually happening, but a consequence of a process that creates them. The constructivist position aims to bring the many constructions that might exist into as much consensus as possible. It does not aim to explain the 'real' world but to show it as it exists at a particular point within a particular set of circumstances. Lincoln (1990) suggests other titles for this particular paradigm, for example 'naturalistic' and 'ethnographic'.

Firestone (1990) feels that these two paradigms have parallels in that they agree at the most basic level about the impossibility of certainty, allowing for a social construction of reality. He feels that where they actually disagree is in terms of how to cope with this, and whereas, at the highest level, the single reality does not appear to equate with the multiple realities of constructivism, these differences are, at an operational level, of degree and emphasis. These ideas suggest a much less distinct boundary between paradigms of research than previous ideas of a completely closed system.

Giddens (1976) suggests that all paradigms are, in fact, mediated by others, believing that:

> The process of learning a paradigm is also a process of learning what a paradigm is not: that is to say, learning to mediate it with other, rejected alternatives by contrast to which, the claims of the paradigm in question are clarified.

Personal beliefs

Beliefs about the world must mediate the researcher's ability to feel comfortable working within different paradigms of research. The process of deciding what particular view of research reflects the researcher's philosophy parallels Giddens' (1976) ideas of learning a paradigm, in that the researcher, rather than positively looking for a philosophy that fits his or her views, tends to discard ideas and concepts until those which are left reflect most closely the researcher's ideas.

In this case, the researcher feels unhappy with the idea of a fixed and immovable 'real world' and a 'truth' that can be discovered, feeling most comfortable with ideas of multiple realities – that what is seen as real is real only at that time and in a particular set of circumstances within the experiences of a particular group of people. This might be summed up as:

> what we take to be objective knowledge and truth is the result of perspective. Knowledge and truth are created, not discovered by mind. (Schwant 1994)

If it is necessary to label these beliefs, the 'best fit' is what many texts describe as a constructivist position.

The aims of this area of research are to provide information about a particular setting with particular circumstances, the views and values of the people involved obviously mediating the enquiry and therefore the results. It should not be necessary therefore to be able to replicate the study in another area, and readers should be able to make decisions about the applicability and transferability of the study from its context and their own values (Lincoln 1990). Lincoln also feels that notions of objectivity are impossible and unnecessary in constructivist research as reality is shaped by values. Firestone suggests, however, that:

> Although one cannot know when truth has been achieved, the warrant for assertions about it can be assessed. The firmest warrant comes from objective inquiry – that is, inquiry that follows the procedures of good research in the field. Objective inquiry may be 'wrong' but it is at least free from gross defects, which should add to one's comfort.

Political considerations must be taken into account when carrying out research in the field of practice, especially if the researcher wishes to have the results noted and acted upon. Although it may feel quite uncomfortable for the researcher, ideas of research may need to be compromised, as health service research, mirroring the tradition of medical research, is often concerned with hard facts rather than with pure descriptions of situations, which tend to be trivialized and ignored. These considerations may, on occasion, lead to a mediation in the research design in order to provide the necessary 'facts' to obtain a validation of and action upon the findings of the research.

The ideas about the area for research and the discussions that surround it are, owing to the nature of research within a practice setting, quite personal to the researcher, although many of the issues are shared by the small team of practitioners who will have an input into the research.

Methodology

After a consideration of the types of data needed in order to explore the aims of the research, a valid approach would seem to be that of the 'triangulation' approach suggested by Goodwin and Goodwin (1984), who felt that a method combining both a qualitative approach looking at opinions and feelings, and a quantitative approach exploring more concrete data, could strengthen the comprehensiveness and validity of a study.

There is no simple question identified in this piece of research where yes/no answers will suffice, but a complex, dynamic situation, mediated by nurses' personal experiences and skills. A broad picture of the situation is needed, and the researcher feels that this may best be found by the use of diverse methods. The range of aims identified in order to explore this multifaceted situation suggest the need to use a variety of approaches.

The most obvious way to examine what conditions and problems are discussed (aim 1) is to look at the documentary evidence already available, a technique often known as secondary data analysis. Each telephone conversation about a patient, either a self-referral (the patient's referral of him- or herself) or a referral by another health professional, is recorded, including the information gained from the referrer and the advice given. This is therefore a good source of information about the patient problems that present by telephone. A large amount of data is collected about patients who actually attend the ophthalmic A&E setting. Some of these, such as what area the patient comes from, are associated with contracting and revenue issues. Other information, for example name, age and address, helps in the recording of episodes and activity. Some information, such as the diagnosis, is recorded partly for completeness, but also as a resource for possible research. Little of the data is computerized.

Although this method of data collection might be described as 'quantitative', the information gathered will be in terms of diagnoses and symptoms, and therefore might better be dealt with by simple descriptive strategies rather than more traditional statistical methods.

A similar argument may be used for the data collected in order to fulfil the second aim of the research. As previously noted, information about the ultimate diagnosis of the patient's problem is recorded for all patients. A telephone triage form is used on which the practitioner records details of the information obtained by telephone. This includes the patient's name, age, signs and symptoms, and a provisional diagnosis or tentative idea of what the problem might be, based on the information given. These two pieces of information – the provisional and ultimate diagnoses – may be matched up for each patient who attends the department, and inferences drawn about the accuracy of the conclusions arrived at by the practitioner, based on the information that is elicited by telephone. The provisional 'diagnosis' is not likely to be completely accurate in many cases as it is based on incomplete information, but it should be possible for the researcher to decide whether the two diagnoses are linked in any significant way.

It would be very easy to interpret the correlation of diagnoses using statistical methods, but although these would give an easy-to-understand and straightforward picture, this would not be the 'whole' story. Symptoms are often documented rather than a 'diagnosis', and the decision about any correlation between these and the final diagnosis must rest on the interpretation of the researcher. Comments about individual incidents may help to highlight certain points, and the results of this will therefore be presented in a simple graphical form, accompanied by descriptive analysis.

The third aim developed because, although on most occasions the practitioner is happy to accept the patient for urgent treatment on the basis of the information gained from the patient or the health professional, other options are also available. When giving advice to a patient, the practitioner may suggest that the patient visit a GP or optometrist, or may reassure the patient that the signs and symptoms either will subside or are innocuous. If a health professional such as a

GP or optometrist is seeking advice, the practitioner may suggest treatment or investigations, that the patient is referred by the optometrist to the GP (or vice versa), or that the patient is referred routinely to the outpatient department rather than as an emergency. In all these situations, the practitioner must rely on information gained by questioning, and if this information is incomplete, there is the possibility of incorrect advice being offered. This scenario is worrying for all practitioners as, particularly in the case of eye problems, a delay in the management of some problems can lead to serious long-term sequelae.

The only way to determine whether potentially sight-threatening conditions are being diverted away from the emergency service would seem to be to look at what we decide *not* to accept. Various methods for doing this might be considered. A telephone call made to the patient, or a questionnaire sent to the patient (or health professional) to ask him or her what eventually happened, has major ethical and practical implications. Neither patient nor health professional is likely to be happy to co-operate with a researcher if emergency consultation has been refused, especially if the delay in management has in fact led to further problems.

One solution might actually be to accept a number of patients who, based on the information obtained by telephone, would normally not be accepted but instead either reassured or have other strategies suggested to them. This might also pose some ethical, as well as logistical, problems, but GPs and optometrists are likely to be happy with the fact that their patient is being accepted, even when they are informed that he or she would not normally have been accepted, if they know that the effectiveness of telephone triage is being evaluated. Patients are, in the researcher's experience, likely to feel the same. It might be felt that it would be easier not to explain the anomalous acceptance of patients either to them or to other health-care professionals, but this might lead to unrealistic expectations of the service in the future and is, in effect, a 'dishonest' way of obtaining the data.

After experiencing the role of the practitioner undertaking telephone triage and examining some of the telephone triage records, it is quite obvious that patients are accepted into the service who do not match the acceptance criteria and would not normally be accepted. This may be caused by a variety of reasons. One common one is that pressure to accept the patient is exerted on the practitioner by the health-care professional, more usually a GP than an optometrist, although the latter situation also occurs. The practitioner finds it very difficult to refuse to accept a patient if the health-care professional actually insists and will not take no for an answer. Other situations also arise when the patient is accepted even though the presenting features suggest that he or she should not be. These include anomalies in the outpatient system that would mean an excessive wait for a routine or even a more urgent appointment, or where patients have particular personal circumstances or health problems and the practitioner decides to accept them even though the situation does not fulfil the criteria.

In the Emergency Eye Centre, patients who have, in theory, been denied access to the service and have received information about their condition or a more appropriate form of referral are still at liberty to attend. If they do so, the service has an obligation to examine them and treat, advise or refer them as necessary. This situation means that a number of patients attend when the practitioner is happy that they should not. Once these patients have been examined and a definitive diagnosis arrived at, the telephone information may be correlated with the actual consultation information to examine whether or not the initial decision to deny the patient access to the emergency service was correct, or whether it would have been modified in the light of the subsequent information.

A further possible method for one subset of clients would be to correlate the findings at the first routine outpatient appointment with the telephone triage sheet, when this method of referral was that suggested to the referrer. A further investigation of this method, however, suggested that practical considerations would make its adoption impossible. There tended to be a lack of information on telephone triage sheets about the patients who should have been referred for routine outpatient appointments by GPs. Because of the vast number of patients attending the hospital, a significant amount of data – including name, address and date of birth – is needed to positively identify a particular patient, and some of this information, usually the address, was inevitably lacking on the telephone triage sheet. This avenue was thus not pursued.

A further method of checking on the decision not to accept a patient was, however, devised. A significant number of patients and health-care professionals are happy to be given advice on conditions and treatments by telephone, and are advised that should any problems occur, or they have any worries, they should, in the case of health-care professionals, contact the service again or, in the case of patients, attend the Emergency Eye Centre. These triage records were kept, and the records for the following week checked to discover whether further contact had been made or the patient had attended. If no further contact had been made, it was assumed that the information or advice had been all that was necessary and that the triage decision not to accept was correct. A week may seem quite an arbitrary timescale, but ophthalmic conditions tend to progress quite quickly and may be painful. If the triage decision was wrong, practitioners felt that the patient would attend, or further contact would be made, in a matter of 1 or 2 days, so that after a week, it might be assumed that the triage decision and advice given had been correct.

In order to decide on the most useful method by which to examine the practitioners' decision-making, it is useful to consider the views of writers interested in this area. Benner (1984) argues that expert practitioners view situations holistically, drawing on past concrete experience in order to make a decision, whereas the merely proficient must use conscious problem-solving. She feels that this knowledge is embedded in practice. Meerabeau (1992) suggests that:

> if expert knowledge is tacit, it cannot be researched by exclusively verbal methods such as questionnaires; open ended discussion may be appropriate, or perhaps participant observation.

Meerabeau feels that open-ended discussion may facilitate reflection, and that the interaction with other practitioners may help to uncover 'hidden' meanings, motivations and methods of decision-making that would remain 'hidden' if simple questionnaires were used, although she goes on to suggest that findings will not be neatly or easily analysed.

Although questionnaires are a convenient method of data collection and can be formulated to include both qualitative and quantitative data, they cannot, by their very nature, provide a particularly large amount of space for the 'subjects' to enlarge on their own experiences. The researcher is not able to explore particular areas in any further detail, as the questionnaire is usually filled in without the researcher being present and, as a single subject is involved, no discussion can take place. Without accepting Benner's conclusions about expert knowledge being, to some extent, tacit, the researcher feels that this possibility must be allowed for in the research design.

Because a greater exploration of the decision-making process would be necessary than would be allowed by questionnaires, Meerabeau's suggestion of participant observation might provide more useful information. Discussion might take place immediately after a telephone consultation in order to examine the process of decision-making that took place. In order to do this most effectively, the conversation could be tape-recorded so that the subject could remember what had been said and be able to follow the decision-making path. Unfortunately, it is not easily possible to audiotape both sides of a telephone conversation, and even if it were possible, there are ethical considerations such as consent by the client to the conversation being recorded, which, if it were obtained, might lead to a distortion of the conversation because of the awareness that this was happening.

A further method – the one that will be undertaken in these particular circumstances – is a small group or individual structured interview with practitioners soon after telephone triage. A number of cases might be discussed in detail, the discussion between the practitioners, and the exploration of the procedure by more than one practitioner, possibly leading to the discovery of common ideas and feelings about the decision-making process. After considering the advantages and disadvantages of other methods, this is the method that seems most likely to provide useful information. There are only a small number of practitioners in this area; all know each other and work closely as colleagues and members of the same nursing 'team'. Thus, problems of interaction and a lack of 'safety', which might be an issue if the discussion took place between relative strangers, are not likely to cause significant difficulties.

The interpretation of the information generated by these group interviews is identified by Miller and Crabtree (1994) as an iterative process:

> the analysis approach often changes through the collection/analysis cycles and needs to remain open to emergent experience and design.

Having identified the methods for acquiring the data in order to satisfy the aims of the research, the actual process of data collection and analysis may proceed. Each of the research aims was considered separately with regard to issues of data collection.

The A&E service is used by up to 17 000 new patients annually. Because of constraints of time and resources, it was not feasible to expect to include all these patients in the part of the study undertaken to examine what conditions present to the department or are discussed with nurses undertaking telephone triage. A more manageable convenience sample was used of patients presenting over the period of 1 month. This might include up to 1400 new patient episodes in the Emergency Eye Centre alone – a significant number that should show a variety of diagnoses with a spread that might be considered not too dissimilar from that obtained for all patients presenting.

The second aim of the research was met by a subpopulation analysis of the same group used to examine the diagnoses, that is, the same 1-month sample. The telephone triage record was to be examined and correlated with the available actual diagnosis. The number of records in this case was much reduced as most patients present to the Emergency Eye Centre without telephoning first, and nurse practitioner referrals, which make up a significant proportion of the workload of the ARC, are not telephone triaged. Three hundred and three telephone triage records were examined from the ARC, and 158 from the Emergency Eye Centre.

The same time period and telephone triage records were used for the collection of data relating to patients who were triaged as not needing urgent referral. The provisional diagnosis of those patients who were accepted for various reasons, even though it was not felt that their condition warranted urgent assessment, was examined in conjunction with the final diagnosis to ascertain whether the decision to deny access would have been correct. In those instances when advice was given, ARC and Emergency Eye Centre records were checked for the following week to determine whether the patient actually attended or whether more advice or an appointment was sought. If not, the telephone triage decision to give advice only or to deny access was assumed to be correct.

The fourth aim of the research involved small group and individual structured interviews by the researcher with the six nurse practitioners who were all willing to participate in the study. A descriptive analysis of these interviews was undertaken.

Confidentiality

Confidentiality is an issue when patients are involved, but this does not need to cause a problem here. There is no reason why, using any of the methodologies described, a patient should be identified. Certainly, if the particular time of data collection is not noted, the identification of individual patients will be completely impossible. The nurses involved in the study are not named, and all were asked to participate on this basis.

Bias

'Bias' is an issue in all research and is probably inevitable when the researcher is part of the research setting. There are advantages and drawbacks to the researcher being so closely linked to the area of research. Lawler (1991) suggests that it requires an insider to appreciate the nuances being discussed, but that knowledge of the setting may also mean that there are features of practice best researched by an 'outsider'. However, only by being inside the situation can it be truly understood, and it becomes much harder to describe because there is much more to take into consideration than might be realized by someone researching outside the situation. In this case, there is little choice in the matter. The aims of this research are to gain information about a particular setting with particular circumstances, and the views and values of the people involved will obviously affect the enquiry, and therefore the results. It should not be necessary to replicate the study in another area, and the reader should be able to make decisions about the applicability and transferability of the study from its context and his or her own values (Lincoln 1990). Others may interpret the data differently in the same situation, and certainly, in different areas, the same sort of information, interpreted in the light of local circumstances, might lead to different conclusions.

It might be felt that a study of any group of equivalently trained nurses would probably give equivalent results. The study is temporally grounded, however, because of the specific group of nurses targeted in this case, each bringing their unique professional and personal experiences to the role of the nurse practitioner. It is thus unlikely that this study would be replicable, but the view of the researcher is that this is not what is intended of the research, which is to examine *this* particular setting at *this* particular time. Some results may be of interest to or of use in other settings, but the overall picture is unique.

Chapter 3
Presentation of data

Aim 1: To examine what problems present to the department

A sample of 1 month's records was examined. The results were divided into appropriate groupings for ease of presentation, as the range of problems experienced by patients presenting to the A&E service encompasses a vast range of diverse ophthalmic and more general problems that manifest via ophthalmic symptoms.

The results have been separated into problems presenting to the Emergency Eye Centre and the ARC, and then combined to reflect the overall picture. Patients presenting to the Emergency Eye Centre who are referred to the ARC are recorded in each area to accurately reflect the workload, but this gives a distorted picture of the actual patients, and thus diagnoses, presenting. The combined figure has been adjusted to reflect the true situation.

For example, the number of patients presenting to the Emergency Eye Centre with uveitis was 60, and the number of patients with uveitis treated by the ARC was 68. The total number of patients who were treated for uveitis would therefore seem to be 128. In fact, many of the patients from the Emergency Eye Centre were referred to the ARC for treatment, and a small number were referred to the outpatient department. The actual number of patients who presented with uveitis was 71, although, to accurately reflect the workload, the number of patient episodes must be recorded as 128.

Tables 3.1–3.7 show the number of patients presenting with different problems.

Table 3.1: Patients presenting to the A&E service with inflammatory problems

Condition	Emergency Eye Centre	Acute Referral Centre	Overall
Uveitis	60	68	71
Posterior uveitis	–	1	1
Panuveitis	–	1	1
Blepharitis	32	10	37
Marginal keratitis	20	10	21
Episcleritis	11	8	11
Allergy	21	7	26
Vernal conjunctivitis	1	–	1
Corneal degeneration	1	–	1

Table 3.2: Patients presenting to the A&E service with infection

Condition	Emergency Eye Centre	Acute Referral Centre	Overall
Conjunctivitis	126	12	131
Chalazion	81	9	86
Corneal ulcer	10	13	15
Herpes simplex	10	23	24
Disciform keratitis	6	3	6
Herpes zoster	2	9	10
Keratitis	9	4	10
Orbital cellulitis	1	1	1
Preseptal cellulitis	2	3	3
Dacryocystitis	2	2	2
Lid abscess	–	1	1
Ophthalmia neonatorum	–	1	1
Acne rosacea	–	1	1

Table 3.3: Patients presenting to the A&E service with trauma

Condition	Emergency Eye Centre	Acute Referral Centre	Overall
Abrasion	187	22	204
Recurrent abrasion	24	4	26
Conjunctival abrasion	8	–	8
Insect bite	1	–	1
Corneal foreign body	149	5	152
Subtarsal foreign body	31	–	31
Other foreign body	3	–	3
Chemical burns	56	13	59
Welding flash (UV burn)	13	1	14

(cont)

Table 3.3 cont

Condition	Emergency Eye Centre	Acute Referral Centre	Overall
Corneal burn	3	1	4
Plaster cast (lid burns)	1	–	1
Keratitis(contact lens induced)	14	1	14
Exposure keratitis	6	2	8
Conjunctival laceration	6	1	6
Lid laceration	4	1	5
Facial laceration	1	1	1
Blunt trauma	7	10	11
Traumatic uveitis	9	10	10
Hyphaema	2	7	7
Traumatic mydriasis	–	1	1
Commotio retinae	4	4	4
Blow-out fracture	–	1	1
Facial fracture	1	–	1
Orbital trauma	–	1	1
Orbital airgun pellet	1	1	1

Table 3.4: Patients presenting to the A&E service with postoperative problems

Condition	Emergency Eye Centre	Acute Referral Centre	Overall
Corneal sutures	40	5	44
Graft problems	5	1	5
Cataract problems	7	4	7
Other postoperative problems	9	7	14

Table 3.5: Patients presenting to the A&E service with neurological problems

Condition	Emergency Eye Centre	Acute Referral Centre	Overall
Nerve palsy	6	4	8
Retrobulbar neuritis/optic neuritis	5	6	7
Toxic amblyopia	1	1	1
Papilloedema	2	1	2
Cerebrovascular accident	1	2	2
Trigeminal neuralgia	1	–	1
Unknown neurological problem	2	–	2

Table 3.6: Patients presenting to the A&E service with posterior segment problems

Condition	Emergency Eye Centre	Acute Referral Centre	Overall
Posterior vitreous detachment	16	23	28
Retinal detachment	10	10	10
Central/branch vein occlusion	5	8	8
Central retinal artery occlusion	4	3	4
Floaters	1	1	2
Retinal lesion	1	1	1
Subretinal neovascular membrane	1	4	4
Vitreous haemorrhage	5	5	7
Macular degeneration	1	2	2
Macular hole	–	4	4
Diabetic retinopathy	1	4	4
Retinitis	–	1	1
Disciform maculopathy	1	1	1
Abnormal disc	–	1	1
Age-related macular degeneration	1	4	4
Transient ischaemic attack	2	3	3
Retinal holes	–	1	1
Papillitis	–	1	1
Retinoschisis	–	1	1
Chorioretinal atrophy	–	1	1
Central serous retinopathy	2	–	2

Table 3.7: Patients presenting to the A&E service with various problems

Condition	Emergency Eye Centre	Acute Referral Centre	Overall
Nil found	67	27	84
Dry eyes	64	5	69
Subconjunctival haemorrhage	28	8	33
Migraine	10	4	11
Trichiasis	42	3	45
Lid lesions	2	4	4
Concretions	2	2	4
Chronic open angle glaucoma	5	11	13

(cont)

Table 3.7 cont

Condition	Emergency Eye Centre	Acute Referral Centre	Overall
Lid malposition	3	2	4
Painful blind eye	2	1	2
Spontaneous hyphaema	1	1	1
Refractive problem	4	9	12
Lid swelling	1	1	1
Dermoid	–	1	1
Sub/acute glaucoma	–	4	4
Temporal arteritis	–	1	1
Allergic dermatitis	–	1	1
Cataract	–	1	1
Corneal degeneration/dystrophy	1	4	4
Posterior capsule thickening	5	–	5
Eczema	1	–	1
Alopecia	1	–	1
Lash in punctum	1	–	1
Unknown eye problem	–	1	1

Aim 2: To examine the accuracy of the tentative diagnosis

The two areas (ARC and Emergency Eye Centre) that make up the A&E service have very different patterns of referral. The ARC accepts all patients via telephone referrals from health-care professionals – GPs, optometrists, medical staff from other hospitals, usually general A&E departments and nurse practitioners – with a small number of self-referrals from patients with recurrent problems. The Emergency Eye Centre, however, is a walk-in service that receives a number of referrals by telephone, mainly from patients, asking for advice and wondering whether to attend for treatment, along with a small number of referrals from health professionals. These professional referrals occur at times when the ARC is not open: evenings, weekends and Bank Holidays.

This aim has been fulfilled by correlating the provisional diagnosis or symptoms recorded by the practitioner undertaking telephone triage with the actual diagnosis recorded after the patient has attended the department. Because of the difference in referral patterns to each area, they have been dealt with separately. Nurse practitioner referrals to the the ARC have been excluded. Although nurse practitioners refer a large number of patients to ARC, no telephone triage is actually undertaken on these patients by the practitioner receiving the telephone call.

The categories have been presented graphically in two forms, one graph examining the issue in terms of the actual number of patients involved, and the other in terms of these patients as a percentage of the particular category of referrals, that is, from GPs, optometrists, other hospitals or self-referral.

Acute Referral Centre

The total number of patients attending the ARC who were accepted after telephone triage referral was 243 (Figure 3.1):

- 159 patients were referred by their GPs;
- 38 were referred by optometrists;
- 25 were referred by other hospitals;
- 21 patients self-referred.

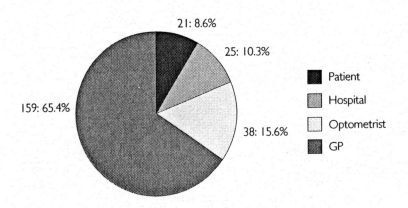

Figure 3.1: ARC – referral pattern (attenders)

A total of 268 patients had been accepted, but 13 – comprising 10 referrals from GPs, 2 from optometrists and 1 from a hospital – did not attend, and 13 forms were so incomplete that information was untraceable.

Of the 125 cases for which a correct provisional diagnosis was arrived at by the nurse, 69 were referred by GPs, 22 by optometrists and 15 from other hospitals, 19 being self-referrals (Figure 3.2). The nurse arrived at a correct provisional diagnosis in 43.4% of all GP referrals, 57.9% of all optometrist referrals, 60% of all patients referred from other hospitals and 90.5% of patient self-referrals (Figure 3.3).

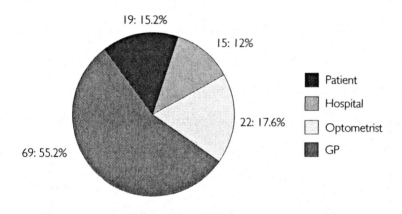

Figure 3.2: ARC – referral pattern of 125 correct provisional diagnoses

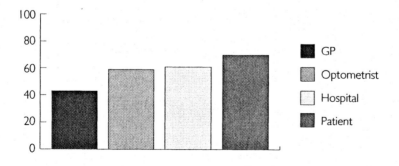

Figure 3.3: ARC – correct provisional diagnosis, percentage of all referrals

Of the 69 GP-referred patients for whom the nurse decided on a correct provisional diagnosis, the GP had also decided upon the correct diagnosis in 34 cases (Figure 3.4). (However, if the 5 patients who were referred to the GP by an optometrist with a correct diagnosis and the 5 patients who knew their own diagnosis are taken into account, this figure reduces to 24.) Of the 22 patients referred by an optometrist, the optometrist had arrived at the correct diagnosis in 16 cases. Of the 15 patients who were referred from hospitals and for whom the nurse had decided on a correct provisional diagnosis, the referrer also had the diagnosis correct in 11 cases. The 19 self-referred patients whose diagnosis was arrived at correctly using telephone triage had all decided on the same diagnosis.

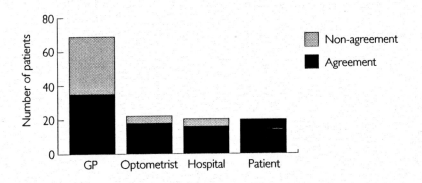

Figure 3.4: ARC – referrer agreement with correct telephone triage diagnosis

Of all patients referred by GPs who were accepted and who attended, the GP was able to decide on a correct diagnosis in 21.4% of cases (Figure 3.5). (This reduces to 15.1% if patients with known diagnoses, referred to the GP by optometrists or self-referred, are discounted.) Optometrists' correct diagnoses made up 42.1% of their referrals, hospital referrals were correct in 44% of cases, and self-referring patients were correct 90.5% of the time.

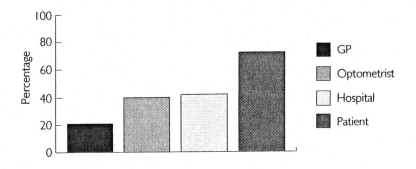

Figure 3.5: ARC – correct referrer diagnosis, percentage of all referrals

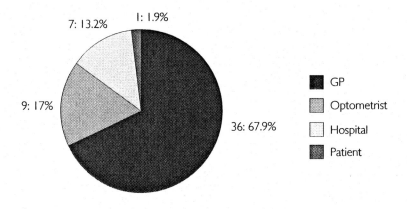

Figure 3.6: ARC – symptoms documented matched final diagnosis well

In 53 cases, the symptoms that were documented matched the final diagnosis well. This figure comprised 36 GP referrals, 9 optometrist referrals, 7 hospital referrals and 1 self-referring patient (Figure 3.6).

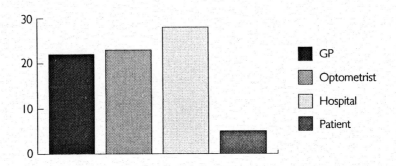

Figure 3.7: ARC – symptoms documented matched diagnosis well, percentage of referrals

The symptoms documented matched the diagnosis well in 22.6% of all GP referrals, 23.7% of all optometrist referrals, 28% of all hospital referrals and 4.8% of patient self-referrals (Figure 3.7).

The symptoms documented or the provisional diagnosis arrived at from the history obtained did not match the eventual diagnosis in 65 cases, made up of 54 GP referrals, 7 optometrist referrals, 3 hospital referrals and 1 self-referral (Figure 3.8).

For patients referred by GPs and who attended, the symptoms recorded or the provisional diagnosis did not match the final diagnosis in 34% of cases (Figure 3.9). This figure was 18.4% for optometrist referrals, 12% for patients referred by hospitals, and 4.8% for self-referred patients.

Emergency Eye Centre

The total number of patients attending who had been referred by telephone was 109 (Figure 3.10):

- 24 patients were referred by GPs;
- 4 were referred by optometrists;
- 12 were referred by other hospitals;
- 69 patients self-referred.

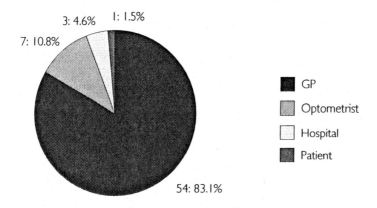

Figure 3.8: ARC – symptoms documented did not match final diagnosis

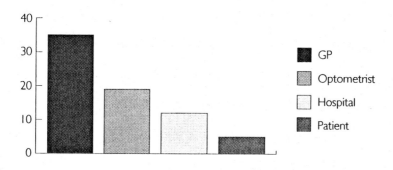

Figure 3.9: ARC – No symptom/diagnosis match, percentage of referrals

A total of 118 patients had been accepted, but 9 did not attend, this figure being made up of 8 patients who self-referred and 1 who had been referred by another hospital.

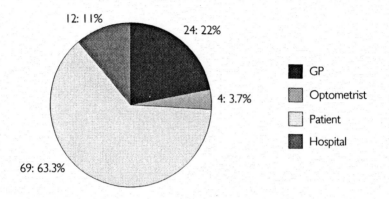

Figure 3.10: Emergency Eye Centre – referral pattern (attenders)

Of the 67 patients for whom a correct provisional diagnosis was arrived at by the nurse (Figure 3.11):

- 12 were referred by GPs;
- 1 was referred by an optometrist;
- 5 were referred by a hospital;
- 49 patients self-referred.

The nurse arrived at the correct provisional diagnosis in 50% of all GP referrals, 25% of all optometrist referrals, 41% of hospital referrals and 71% of all self-referrals by patients (Figure 3.12).

Of the 12 patients for whom the nurse had decided upon a correct provisional diagnosis, the GP had the diagnosis correct in 10 cases (Figure 3.13). The optometrist and nurse agreed on the single correct diagnosis, and the hospital referrer and nurse on all five. Fourteen patients were aware of their own diagnosis, and the nurse identified another 35, giving a total of 49.

Of all patients referred who were accepted and attended, the GPs got 41.7% of the diagnoses correct, the optometrists 25%, the hospital referrers 41.7% and the self-referring patients 20.3% (Figure 3.14).

In 23 cases, the symptoms documented by the nurse matched the final diagnosis well (Figure 3.15).

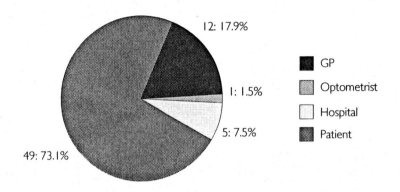

Figure 3.11: Emergency Eye Centre – referral pattern of 67 correct provisional diagnoses

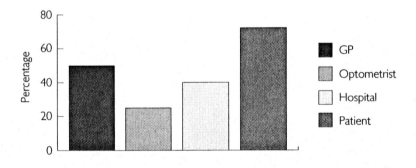

Figure 3.12: Emergency Eye Centre – correct provisional diagnosis, percentage of all referrals

In 25% of GP, optometrist and hospital referrals (a total of 6, 1 and 3 patients respectively) the symptoms documented matched the final diagnosis well (Figure 3.16). Of the patients who self-referred, the figure was 18.8% (13 patients).

In 19 cases, the symptoms documented or the provisional diagnosis did not match the final diagnosis (Figure 3.17). This figure

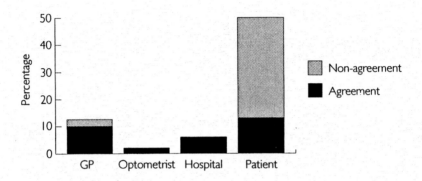

Figure 3.13: Emergency Eye Centre – referrer agreement with correct telephone triage diagnosis

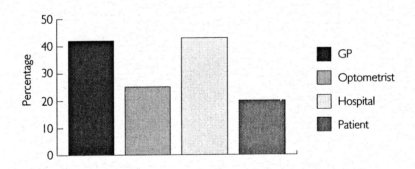

Figure 3.14: Emergency Eye Centre – correct referrer diagnosis, percentage of all referrals

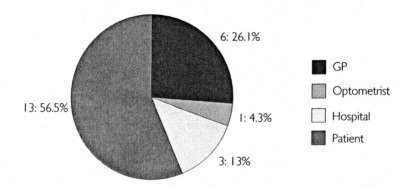

Figure 3.15: Emergency Eye Centre – symptoms documented matched final diagnosis well

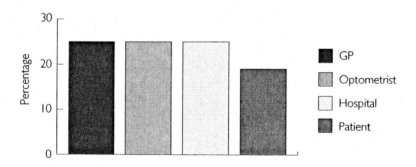

Figure 3.16: Emergency Eye Centre – symptoms documented matched final diagnosis well, percentage of referrals

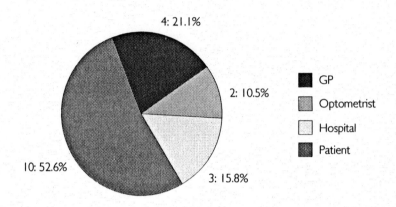

Figure 3.17: Emergency Eye Centre – symptoms documented did not match final diagnosis

is made up of 4 patients from GPs, 2 from optometrists, 3 from other hospitals and 10 patients who self-referred.

In 16.7% of GP referrals (4 patients), the symptoms documented or the provisional diagnosis did not match the final diagnosis (Figure 3.18). This was true for 50% of optometrist referrals (2 patients), 25% of referrals from other hospitals (3 patients) and 14.5% of self-referring patients (10 patients).

The ARC had a very good idea of what patients were expected, that is, where the provisional diagnosis had been correct or the symptoms documented matched the final diagnosis, in (Figure 3.19):

- 66% of patients referred by GPs (105 patients);
- 81.6% of patients referred by optometrists (31 patients);
- 88% of patients referred by other hospitals (22 patients);
- 95.3% of patients who self-referred (20 patients);

giving a total of 73.3% of all patients attending who were referred and accepted by telephone triage.

The Emergency Eye Centre had a very good idea of what patients were expected, that is, where the provisional diagnosis was correct or the symptoms documented matched the final diagnosis of patients who were accepted by telephone triage and attended, in the cases of (Figure 3.20):

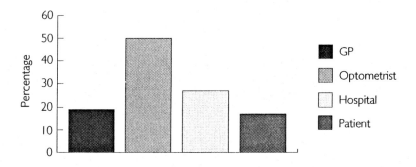

Figure 3.18: Emergency Eye Centre – symptoms documented did not match final diagnosis well, percentage of referrals

- 75% of patients referred by GPs (18 patients);
- 50% of patients referred by optometrists (2 patients);
- 66.7% of patients referred by other hospitals (8 patients);
- 89.8% of patients who self-referred (62 patients);

that is, a total of 82.5% of all patients attending who were referred and accepted by telephone triage.

Because of the small number involved in many of the categories examined, tests of significance are not applicable.

Aim 3: To examine the accuracy of the decision to give urgent treatment

Patients accepted who did not match the acceptance criteria

After the patient has attended, a history has been obtained and a diagnosis has been made, it is obvious that a number of patients would not have been accepted had the nurse been able to obtain an accurate history from the health professional. On a number of occasions, the patient history bears little resemblance to that given by the professional, especially in relation to the timescale, the referrer tending to

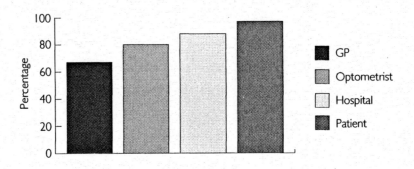

Figure 3.19: Percentage of referrals in which the ARC had a reasonable idea of what patients were expected

give a shorter history than that given by the patient. However, it is not possible to look at these decisions retrospectively.

The main factor prompting the denial of access to the service is a time factor – if the patient has been experiencing the problem for a period of time and will not be harmed by waiting for an outpatient appointment. Most of the referrals with this history were diverted towards routine outpatient appointments. A number of patients with chronic open angle glaucoma were accepted because they had other, more pressing problems. Only two patients with a provisional diagnosis of chronic open angle glaucoma and no other problems were accepted for the ARC, the provisional diagnosis being confirmed after examination.

Patients who, after being given advice, attended anyway

One patient was denied access to the ARC with a provisional diagnosis of dry eyes and was given advice on how to deal with the problem. The patient subsequently attended and was found to have dry eyes.

One patient who telephoned the Emergency Eye Centre gave a history suggesting that the problem was a 'floater' or vitreous opacity, and was reassured and given advice about the situation. The patient

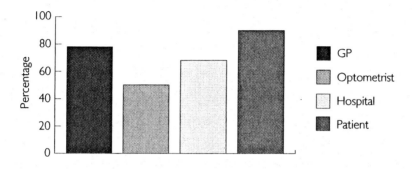

Figure 3.20: Percentage of referrals in which the Emergency Eye Centre had a reasonable idea of what patients were expected

attended the Emergency Eye Centre and was found, after examination, to have a floater. The advice and reassurance were repeated and the patient was discharged.

A further patient telephoned the Emergency Eye Centre and was given advice and education regarding an infected chalazion, for which the correct treatment had already been prescribed by the GP. The patient returned to his GP, who obtained an ARC appointment for him. On examination in the ARC, the diagnosis was confirmed, the treatment remained unchanged, the information and reassurance were reinforced, and the patient was discharged.

Patients who received advice and made no further contact

Of referrals to the ARC, 22 were diverted to an outpatient appointment. Eight were old patients with non-acute problems, referred by both GPs and the patient themselves, and appointments were made for outpatient clinics via the senior medical staff. Eleven patients were referred by the GP and were re-routed to routine outpatient appointments, and in three cases of chronic open angle glaucoma referred by optometrists, staff were asked to send the patient to their GP for referral for a routine outpatient appointment.

Two patients were denied access to the service and were not re-routed. One was not happy with his local eye unit and wished to have a second opinion; the other had missed an appointment at his local eye unit in Cork and wished to come for a 'check-up'.

Twelve referrers were given advice rather than an appointment, and the patients subsequently did not attend. Seven were referred by GPs, one by an optometrist, one by another hospital, and three patients self-referred.

The conditions that were identified during telephone triage for which information was given included:

- 2 of blepharitis (lid inflammation);
- 2 of chalazion (lid cysts);
- 2 in which the patient or the referrer was worried about the postoperative appearance of the eye;
- 2 of herpes zoster in which the eye was not involved;
- 1 of subconjunctival haemorrhage;
- 1 minor chemical burn;
- 1 allergic reaction;
- 1 in which the optometrist could find nothing wrong but the patient was worried as he had a past history of corneal ulcers.

With regard to the Emergency Eye Centre, six patients were advised to attend their GP for referral via the outpatient system as they had very long (up to 2-year) histories of their problems. One optician was advised to refer his patient to a GP for the same reason. Two patients were found on questioning to have no real eye problem (1 having been assaulted and 1 being unwell) and these were referred to local A&E units. Three patients were diverted to more local eye units because they were their convenient for them or, in one case, because the patient was already a patient at that unit.

Advice was given to 22 referrers, and the patients did not subsequently attend or recontact the unit. This figure was made up of 1 patient referred by a GP, 2 by other hospitals and 18 patients self-referring. The doctor referring from another hospital was advised about the treatment of patients with a minor chemical injury and an abrasion. The GP was advised about treatment for a patient with a chalazion.

Patients were given advice, reassurance and health education about the following:

- recurrent erosion (1);
- abrasion (the patient having already been treated elsewhere) (2);
- welding flash (UV light burn) (1);
- eyedrop problems (2);
- chalazion (1);
- blepharitis (1);
- dry eyes (1);
- conjunctivitis (2);
- subconjunctival haemorrhage (3);
- allergy (2);
- problems after a skull fracture (1);
- a glancing blow to the side of the head with no eye problem (1).

Aim 4: To explore the nurses' decision-making process

The nature of the data obtained by interviewing nurse practitioners about their telephone triage decision-making is such that it is best included by description and comment, being integrated into the final chapter of this dissertation.

Chapter 4
Discussion

An examination of the data obtained from 1 month's records of patients presenting to the Emergency Eye Centre and the ARC – which make up the A&E service at Manchester Royal Eye Hospital – shows a vast range of presenting problems, covering the whole spectrum of ophthalmic problems and including other problems that impinge on areas of specialization, for example neurological and vascular problems.

In the Emergency Eye Centre, minor problems predominate. A consideration of a list of the most minor problems presenting to both areas (blepharitis, allergy, conjunctivitis, chalazion, abrasion, foreign body, welding flash, contact lens and exposure keratitis, dry eyes, subconjunctival haemorrhage and concretions) shows that these problems account for 59.3% of patients presenting to the Emergency Eye Centre (765 patients) and 17.1% of those presenting to the ARC (83 patients).

A further consideration of what these 'minor' problems actually are reveals that many of them are extremely painful (abrasion, welding flash and keratitis), while others can be intensely irritating (blepharitis, foreign bodies, dry eyes, allergies and concretions), give rise to worrying symptoms of redness, stickiness and soreness (conjunctivitis) or be visually startling (subconjunctival haemorrhage and allergy).

Although these may be 'minor' conditions when considered by nurse or medical ophthalmic specialists, they are causing the patient problems that need to be resolved. The fact that patients are also referred by health professionals to the ARC with these problems suggests that neither are they 'minor' to many health professionals, who obviously feel that the best way of treating these patients is by referring to a specialist centre.

A proportion of patients were not found to have any ophthalmic problem, this figure being remarkably consistent whether the patient had self-referred or had been referred by a health professional. In the Emergency Eye Centre, the proportion of patients found not to have any ophthalmic problem was 5.2% (67 patients), and in the ARC 5.6% (27 patients). Again, it must be acknowledged that had the patients not felt that they had a problem causing them anxiety, they would not have presented to the service. A successful outcome of care must be measured in terms of resolving anxiety as well as resolving physical ophthalmic problems.

It is clear that the Emergency Eye Centre provides a service for postoperative patients, particularly those needing the removal of corneal sutures after cataract extraction. These patients made up 3% of the workload – 40 patients. One per cent of the ARC workload (five patients) also involved the removal of corneal sutures, but four of these were corneal graft sutures, which are not within the remit of the nurse practitioner in the Emergency Eye Centre.

Having examined the more 'minor' problems presenting to the service, it can be seen that 419 patients presenting to the Emergency Eye Centre (32.4%) had more significant ophthalmic problems, ranging from major infection, inflammatory problems and more major trauma, to neurological problems including raised intercranial pressure and posterior segment problems. All of these problems needed medical examination, most needed intervention, either acutely or in the long run, some needed referral to more appropriate medical specialities, and many needed long-term follow-up. Many of these patients were referred to the ARC, and the range of ophthalmic presentations is matched by that shown by the patients referred to the ARC by health professionals.

It can be seen therefore that, overall, a total of 1522 patients were cared for by the A&E service. A vast range of ophthalmic and other medical problems were experienced by these patients, who were assessed, examined, treated and referred by both nurse practitioners and medical staff working within the service.

The second research aim, in its most simple form, has been quite easily fulfilled by the research. The positive correlation between triage diagnosis and actual diagnosis was found to be 51.4% in the ARC and 61.5% in the Emergency Eye Centre.

Although it was felt initially that the secondary data analysis of the telephone triage sheets would be quite straightforward, it was actually found to be highly complex. Many more variables needed to be taken into account, and the researcher felt unable to be bound by the constraints of the aim as more areas of interest were highlighted. Other areas were therefore also explored in order to give a greater depth of knowledge and understanding of referral patterns to both areas of the A&E departments, and to highlight some of the problems and anomalies surrounding referral, thus uncovering more of the 'whole story'.

During the analysis of the telephone triage records, it was found that, on many occasions, the nurse practitioner did not actively state a provisional diagnosis, but recorded a collection of symptoms or observations and made the decision to accept or deny access on the basis of these. The researcher felt that to exclude all these records on the basis that no provisional diagnosis had been recorded would detract from the true picture of whether the nurse was making effective decisions to accept or deny the patient access to the service based on the information elicited from the telephone call.

By recording symptoms, the nurse had built up a picture of the patient's problem that, on occasion, pointed to only one possible provisional diagnosis, even though the final step of recording a provisional diagnosis had not been taken. This might be for a variety of reasons: the nurse may not feel happy to commit herself to such a concrete statement, feeling happier to work with a small range of possibilities suggested by the symptoms rather than being incorrect about the final, pinpointed diagnosis. Time might also be a factor. The departments are often busy, and the final step might be constrained by the time available to commit to just one of a range of possibilities. Whatever the reason, the documented history was felt by the researcher to be valid in terms of the departments having an idea of what problems patients were likely to present with. The researcher thus felt that these should be included, in a separate category – where the symptoms documented matched the final diagnosis well. This category comprised 21.8% of ARC referrals who were accepted and attended, and 21.1% of Emergency Eye Centre referrals.

These figures are based on the fact that the researcher has a background in the speciality and was able to correlate symptoms with eventual diagnosis. This correlation was only deemed to exist where the link between symptoms and diagnosis was particularly strong. It was not accepted merely if a vague link existed. This might be seen to be a very subjective exercise, but an experience of the speciality and of the presenting signs and symptoms of patients with particular problems led, the researcher feels, to objectivity, which was strengthened by the application of random checks of the perceived correlations by ophthalmic specialist colleagues.

The proportions of patients in this category – where the symptoms documented matched the final diagnosis well – led to an overall picture of the staff's knowledge of referrals. The ARC staff had a reasonable idea of the problems experienced by 73.3% of the patients whom they were expecting, and the Emergency Eye Centre 82.5% of them.

These high figures suggest that the questioning techniques employed by the nurse practitioners and the decisions made on the basis of the telephone triage consultation are of very high quality. This does not reflect the results of Crouch's (1992) study, which found that when nurses in general A&E departments were undertaking telephone triage, questioning was poor and decisions were made hastily and without the full facts. However, much telephone triage in other areas is performed on an ad hoc basis (Glasper 1993), and in the Manchester Royal Eye Hospital departments, telephone triage has been formalized, is of major importance to the smooth running of the areas, and is carried out by experienced personnel, as Wheeler (1989) suggests should be the case.

The group of patients in whom the symptoms documented did not match the eventual diagnosis was felt by the researcher to be of great interest, and the reasons for this lack of agreement were explored. Of patients referred to the ARC, there were 65 cases (26.7%) in which the symptoms documented did not match the final diagnosis, this figure being 19 cases (17.4%) for the Emergency Eye Centre.

On further investigation, the reasons for the poor history reflected the referrer of the patient. Of the patients referred to ARC in whom a poor history was obtained, 1.5% (1 patient; 4.8% of self-referrals) self-referred by giving a diagnosis of what he thought was happening to his eye (a corneal melt, which he had been warned might happen). He was very anxious about the possibility, and it was impossible to obtain a good history because of this. Of the other referrals, 4.6% (3 patients) came from other hospitals (12% of hospital referrals), and all cases were patients for whom doctors felt that what was eventually diagnosed as a refractive error was actually a blurring as a side-effect of the drugs being taken by the patient. Nearly 11% (10.8%) of the referrals (7 patients) were from optometrists (18.4% of optometrist referrals), who generally give an excellent history that is accepted with little question by the triage nurse. In these cases, the optometrist was mistaken in his assessment of the situation.

The greatest majority of patients, 83.1% (54 patients), were referred by GPs, a figure that far outweighs the proportion of patients referred by GPs to ARC (65.4%) and is a total of 34% of all GP referrals. A further investigation of these triage sheets revealed that, in some cases, the GP assumed that the problem was similar to one which the patient had experienced before and did not examine other possibilities. In a number of cases, the GP had made a definite diagnosis, which he gave to the nurse practitioner (and which was in fact incorrect), and was reluctant, in some cases actually refusing, to discuss the symptoms and condition of the patient with the triage nurse, leading to an incorrect provisional diagnosis. A number of patients attending from GPs were found to have no eye problem, particularly in cases of assault and herpes zoster (shingles), the GP feeling that a 'check-up' was appropriate. Other cases included one for whom history elicited from the GP was not reflected in the letter sent by him with the patient and, on occasion, where patients presented with a history different from that given by the GP and were found to have a chronic rather than an acute problem.

In the Emergency Eye Centre, the number and proportion of patients were much smaller: 17.4% (19 patients). In this case, by far the largest category was that of self-referring patients (10 patients; 52.6% of this category and 14.5% of all self-referring patients). Most of these patients felt that they had an eye problem, although this could not be substantiated by examination. A great deal of reassurance was needed to satisfy these patients. Of the referrals, 21.1% were from GPs (4 patients; 16.7% of GP referrals), a figure much less than that experienced in ARC. Referrals from GPs to the Emergency Eye Centre only happen outside normal working hours, and patients tend to present to GPs with more acute and obvious problems during this time; thus, the proportion of incorrect diagnoses is likely to be less. Two patients from optometrists (50% of optometrist referrals) did not have matching provisional and final diagnoses. Again, this is because of the fact that the nurse tends to accept the optometrist's diagnosis, if presented with one, with little question, as optometrists are perceived to have an excellent ophthalmic knowledge. The three patients from other hospital (15% of the sample, equal to 25% of hospital referrals) all had more serious trauma than had been thought by the presenting doctor.

The analysis of the telephone triage records led to an examination of the referral patterns to the ARC and Emergency Eye Centre, and, further, to an examination of patterns of correlation between nurse and referrer diagnoses. In the ARC, patient self-referrals accounted for 8.6% of the total number – 21 patients. As the patients who are able to self-refer are those who have recurrent problems, it is not surprising that the nurse arrived at a correct provisional diagnosis in 90.5% of cases (19) and that the patient agreed with the diagnosis in all these cases.

Medical staff from other hospitals accounted for 10.3% of referrals (25 patients). In 15 cases (60%), the nurse arrived at a correct provisional diagnosis, and in these, the referrer had come to a correct diagnosis in 11 cases, a total of 44% of referred patients. Nearly all of these patients were referred from general A&E departments and had obvious minor trauma and good patient histories, enabling the correct diagnosis by the referrer. The nurse was enabled by the history to make a correct provisional diagnosis in a further three cases.

Optometrists referred 38 patients (15.6% of the total), a correct provisional diagnosis being arrived at for 22 patients – 57.9% of optometrist referrals. Of these 22, the optometrist had arrived at a correct diagnosis in 16 cases, equalling 42.1% of referrals. It might be expected that the figure would be higher considering the optometrist's background and knowledge of ophthalmic problems. However, many of the patients referred by optometrists had complex problems, particularly retinal problems, about which it is very difficult to come to a diagnostic conclusion. The nurse practitioners who were interviewed had a very positive view of optometrist referrals, one going as far as to say:

> Opticians are wonderful – they really are wonderful.
> They know what they're looking at – it's their forte.

Referrals from GPs accounted for 65.4% of referrals to the ARC: 159 patients. The telephone conversation led to the nurse arriving at a correct provisional diagnosis in 69 cases, accounting for only 43.4% of all GP referrals. Of these 69 patients, the GP had a correct diagnosis in 34 cases (21.4% of all GP referrals). This figure is further reduced because of those patients who referred themselves to their GP and knew their own diagnosis because it was a recurrent problem (5 patients), as well as the 5 patients who were referred to their GP by an optometrist who gave the GP the correct diagnosis, which he subsequently passed on to the ARC. Taking this into account, the GPs were able to correctly diagnose only 16.1% of the patients whom they referred to the ARC.

This is obviously a very low figure, reflecting perhaps a lack of ophthalmic knowledge by GPs. One factor in the nurse practitioners' low provisional diagnosis rate seems to be a problem with the history elicited from the GP. Many of the patient histories obtained when the patient arrived were noticeably different from those given by the GP, especially with regard to the severity and duration of the symptoms. It might be suggested that, in some cases, histories are exaggerated in order to obtain an acute appointment when it is not particularly appropriate. A further factor highlighted both by the examination of the telephone triage record sheets and the discussion with the nurse practitioners is the reluctance of the GPs in particular to discuss problems with nurses. Interviews with nurse practitioners led to the conclusion that some GPs have a problem referring a patient to a nurse:

> because we are nurses and not accepted as an individual with specialist knowledge – maybe they feel threatened ... 'Nurse practitioner' is just a title – it isn't, to them, another higher-level professional person who has an in-depth knowledge of ophthalmics and is more likely to have a knowledge far greater then theirs.

Another nurse practitioner felt that:

> some GPs expect you to accept and consider it a personal affront to have to go into all this rigmarole about the state of the eye. Some, I've had to pull it out of them, and some don't tell me at all.

Yet another suggested that some GPs:

> get very angry that you are impertinent enough to
> question their diagnosis of a patient when really all you
> are doing is gathering information together to get a
> provisional diagnosis.

The nurse practitioners felt that the GPs did not like being questioned because:

> it shows up their inadequacies and the fact that they
> might not even have looked at the eye or the patient.

This nurse practitioner also felt, along with others, that GPs are sometimes actively giving misleading information in order to obtain an appointment. When asked whether it was easier to obtain a history from a patient, she said:

> Yes, I have to ask a lot more than with a GP generally. At
> least it's usually truthful; they don't have insights. GPs
> know what things will get them into ARC, whereas the
> patient won't.

Nurse practitioners also felt very pressured by GPs to accept patients, feeling that some displayed aggressive behaviour and/or used emotional blackmail such as 'If it was your mother ...' in order to obtain an appointment.

It would be unfair to label all GPs in this way, but there is a strong perception among nurse practitioners of the differences between what are known as 'good' and 'bad' GPs. The nurses felt that, 'some doctors are delighted that we ask questions and are so pleased to get information'. Others felt that GPs were, on the whole, getting better and were more forthcoming with the information needed by the nurse practitioner, one suggesting that if the GPs had taken the trouble to see the patients and collect the symptoms, as well as to make the decision that the patients could not be treated by them, the nurse practitioner might well accept the patients even if they were on the borderline of the criteria for acceptance into the ARC.

The referral pattern for patients seen in the Emergency Eye Centre was found to be totally different from that of the ARC, a finding that had been expected. Referrals from GPs accounted for only 22% of referrals (24 patients), and in half of these, the nurse decided on a correct provisional diagnosis. The GP made the same decision in 10 out of the 12 patients, equal to 41.7% of their referrals. One of these patients had recurrent problems, and another was referred by an optometrist to the GP. The collection of symptoms from GPs was also better, leading to the department being aware of what patients were expected in 75% of patients referred from GPs. This may reflect that many of calls were out of normal working hours, and patients were presenting with more acute and easily recognized problems.

Referrals from optometrists accounted for 3.7% of patients, a total of only four patients. Only one provisional diagnosis was correct, and a further single patient's symptoms matched the final diagnosis; thus, the EEC was aware of what was likely to be presenting in only 50% of optometrist referrals. However, this amounted to only four patients, a fairly insignificant number. Of the two patients whose symptoms did not match the diagnosis, one was thought to have a visual field defect, although this proved not to be the case on examination, and the other presented to the optometrist with a sudden loss of vision, which could not in fact have been sudden as it was found to be caused by refractive error. Hospital referrals to the Emergency Eye Centre totalled 12, 11% of the total. The provisional diagnosis was correct for five patients, and the referrer had the correct diagnosis in all these cases. A further three patients' symptoms matched the final diagnosis, an overall agreement of 66.7%. The other four patients' histories were presented incompletely by the referrer.

Patient referrals made up 63.3% of Emergency Eye Centre referrals, 69 patients in total. Of these, 73.1% (49 patients) were accorded a correct provisional diagnosis. In only 14 cases (20.3%) were patients actually aware of their own diagnosis, for example that they had an abrasion, a foreign body or a recurrent problem, in contrast with 100% of those referring to the ARC. In the vast majority of these cases, the nurse made a correct decision based on information gained from the patient. A further 13 patients' documented symptoms matched the final diagnosis, leading to the Emergency Eye Centre staff having a reasonable idea of what patients were expected in a total of 89.8% of telephone triaged patient self-referrals.

The interviews with nurse practitioners again suggested some reasons for the ability of the nurse to come to the correct conclusion. Most nurse practitioners felt that it was sometimes difficult to obtain a history from a patient because the information given was much more vague, but that the history was eventually much better and more complete. One nurse practitioner felt that, on the whole, GPs were the easiest group from which to obtain a history, although:

> a bad GP is as bad as a poor historian patient, and worse because a poor historian patient won't get annoyed with you and won't assume they have a knowledge ... you can still keep digging and they don't get upset or temperamental but will continue to answer questions the best they can.

Another nurse practitioner felt that the history often had to be 'dragged out' of the patient, especially if he or she was frightened and anxious. This nurse felt that it was important not to lead patients as they would then tend to answer yes to everything. She felt that the nurse practitioner could ask the patient to look in a mirror in order to describe the eye, and felt that, although it took longer to obtain a history, it was a better history. As previously highlighted, one of the nurse practitioners felt strongly that a history from a patient was likely to be truthful.

Overall, therefore, it seems that the departments have a reasonable idea of the problems that patients who have been accepted via telephone triage are likely to present with in a high proportion of cases: 73.3% of patients accepted by the ARC and 82.5% of patients accepted by the Emergency Eye Centre.

The proportion that does not fall into this category seems often to result from poor histories obtained from referrers, sometimes because of the complexity of the presenting problems, but with a significant proportion of poor histories caused by the reluctance of GPs to discuss patients with an ophthalmic specialist nurse practitioner. Many things affect the telephone triage record and the formation of a provisional diagnosis. The history that the nurse is able to obtain is influenced by the willingness of the referrer to give information. The obtaining of signs and symptoms is a two-way process; however skilled the nurse is in interpreting information and however experienced, the whole picture will not be painted if the referrer is unwilling to give information.

No one expects GPs to have a vast knowledge of ophthalmology, but a willingness to discuss with other professionals seems to be an underlying theme, both within the results obtained by secondary data analysis and in the perceptions of the nurse practitioners who deal with the GPs' telephone calls. It is unfair to include all GPs in the same category, and this has also been highlighted by the nurse practitioners. Many GPs are felt to be happy to discuss problems, to accept advice and therefore obtain the full value of the service.

Nurse practitioners feel that, on the whole, they have a good relationship with optometrists and are able to discuss things at a professional level, as they are with doctors from other hospitals, particularly those from the surrounding A&E departments. The department has links with local A&E departments that are strengthened by regular lectures to new junior doctors. Nurses are able to elicit good histories from patients and are able to make correct provisional diagnoses in a high proportion of these telephone consultations, even when the patient does not have a knowledge or insight into the condition.

The third aim of the research was felt to be particularly important. Although Stetson (1986) has reported that telephone triage is a vital component of problem diagnosis and could save time if performed correctly, and some authors (for example, Kernohan et al 1992, Wilkins 1992) hold telephone triage to be a very positive development, others believe that telephone triage could prove to be a major problem, to the extent that Dunn (1985) has suggested that the rule for responding to telephone information requests should be to tell patients to attend the hospital. According to Glasper (1993):

> imparting nursing information over the telephone is
> analogous to nursing with your eyes closed and your
> hands tied behind your back.

A secondary data analysis of telephone triage records has in fact shown that, in many cases, the information that the nurse is able to obtain over the telephone is useful, aiding the formation of an accurate provisional diagnosis and an awareness of what problems patients are going to present to the department with. The nurse practitioners in both the ARC and the Emergency Eye Centre were very aware of the fact that, on occasion, they offered advice to both patients and referring health professionals as a result of telephone information, and were concerned that the information given was accurate and of use to the referrer, the alternative strategies suggested for treatment or referral not jeopardizing the ophthalmic condition of the patient.

A recent study by Kunkler and Mitchell (1994) in a general A&E department showed that the staff gave correct advice in response to a telephone call about a patient with cardiac pain in 75% of cases. This might be felt to be quite a high proportion but, in fact, shows that 25% of the time the information was incorrect or incomplete, which might cause major problems in a life-threatening situation. The nature of problems presenting to an ophthalmic A&E service is such that life is not likely to be threatened if incorrect information is given, although, of course, sight may be. It was most important to the nurse practitioners, and obviously of concern to the users and managers of the service, to know whether correct and useful information had been given during the telephone triage consultations, and to be as sure as possible that potentially sight-threatening conditions had not been missed.

A number of patients and referrers contacted the service over the period studied and were given advice about the treatment or possible course of a particular condition, or information about other referral strategies. Of the 22 patients who were diverted towards outpatient rather than ARC appointments, 8 were patients with known problems, and it was considered more appropriate that they see their consultant's team urgently rather than the doctor in the ARC. These appointments were intended to be acute or soon, and were left in the control of the registrar or senior registrar.

Several patients were referred by GPs, who were asked to refer by letter to the outpatient department for a routine appointment. These were patients in whom the history was of anything from one month to two years in duration, whose problems were not therefore felt to be acute. The referral letters sent to the hospital are all examined by senior medical staff, who allocate a priority for an appointment based on the information given by the referrer; thus, a more urgent problem should be given an earlier appointments. Optometrists referred a number of patients with a newly diagnosed chronic open angle glaucoma, and were asked to refer to outpatients via the GP. Although this is an important finding, it is felt that the wait for an outpatient appointment will cause no further problem for the patient's visual prognosis, and this has been built into protocols for the acceptance of patients for acute appointments.

A total of 34 referrers were given advice about treatment or reassurance for an eye condition after consideration of the telephone triage history. Problems identified by the nurse practitioner ranged from postoperative problems, allergies and infections, to minor trauma and idiopathic subconjunctival haemorrhage. Instead of following up these patients by telephone, which was felt to be ethically inappropriate, an assumption was made that if the patient or referrer did not re-present to the service for further information or treatment within 1 week, the information given had been valid and appropriate for that patient. This was a massive assumption, but all patients and referrers were informed as a matter of routine that they should contact the service again if they had any problems or were at all worried. Patients who refer to the Emergency Eye Centre are anyway at liberty to attend the service without an appointment, and none of these did, leading to the conclusion that the information given to patients at a telephone triage consultation is valid and safe, which was the major consideration for the nurse practitioners and users of the service.

Some confirmation of the accuracy and safety of this information-giving service was provided by three patients who attended the service having been given information that was felt to obviate the need for attendance. Two patients attended the Emergency Eye Centre, and in each case, the diagnosis arrived at through telephone triage was found to be accurate; the information already supplied was reinforced, and further reassurance was given. One patient attended a GP after having been given treatment advice via the telephone. The GP subsequently obtained an ARC appointment for this patient; again, the diagnosis arrived at and the advice given on telephone triage were found to be accurate, treatment was unchanged, and information was reinforced. This provided confirmation of the accuracy of the information and advice given at the telephone consultation, and reassurance about the validity of telephone advice in general in these areas.

It thus seems that the decision to give advice about the condition is, if not necessarily totally accurate (because it is not possible to be positive about this), at least safe. No patient attended with a diagnosis other than that which the nurse practitioner expected or had given advice for, and no treatment was changed.

In order to fulfil the fourth aim of the research, the nurse practitioners were interviewed individually, and the interviews tape-recorded. It is interesting that the responses to the themes of the interview were quite consistent across the nurse practitioners, who had not apparently discussed the subjects between themselves.

The first discussion was based on how the nurse practitioner makes the decision to accept or deny access on the basis of the telephone call. All the nurse practitioners identified a range of symptoms and signs elicited from the referrer on which they based their decision. On the whole, they then formed a picture of what might be going on – a provisional diagnosis – towards which they geared further questions to confirm or refute their hypothesis. This idea of what was 'going on' was felt to be very much a subconscious one, and the provisional diagnosis was decided upon at slightly different times during the telephone triage conversation. One nurse practitioner stated:

> by the time you've gained a basic set of information from them, you've already half made up your mind what the diagnosis is, and you gauge the rest of your questions to what you think it might already be.

She felt that:

> you give a provisional diagnosis right at the beginning because you need to have some idea as to what you think might be going on so you can design the questions to get out of them more information, and as you get these answers you can alter the hypothesis that you've made.

The decision-making seems to be a dynamic process, and this is echoed by the other nurse practitioners. One felt that she only made an early assumption of a diagnosis if the problem were obvious, but she still organized her questions to:

> go off in a particular direction to come to a conclusion and get a picture of what's going on.

Another nurse practitioner felt that she asked specific questions and came to a potential diagnosis at the end of the conversation. Nurse practitioners identified a strategy of 'getting a picture in their head' and trying to prove or disprove this with questions.

This hypothesis-building strategy strongly echoes the strategies discovered by Edwards (1994), who examined the decision-making processes used by nurse practitioners undertaking telephone triage in another area. He felt that the triage decisions were arrived at within a systematic and identifiable framework, this being confirmed by these interviews, which report that a hypothesis is generated and tested against both further questions and the nurse's knowledge. Tanner et al (1987) also suggested that expert nurses used hypothesis-testing in order to come to a conclusion.

A further theme of the interview was based on perceptions of the difficulties of obtaining information during a telephone conversation with respect to the background of the referrer (GP, optometrist, other hospital doctor or patient), and this has been dealt with elsewhere in the text. This discussion led on to a discussion about the 'triggers' that were identified in the conversations. The nurse practitioners felt that some signs and symptoms acted as a trigger for accepting rather than denying the patient access to the service. These include findings such as excessive pain and recent loss of vision. They felt, however, that some referrers had also learnt the triggers and 'knew what buttons to press', and that this led to patients being accepted who would not have been if an accurate history could have been obtained. The patient's history on presentation was different from that given by the referrer – very noticeably so on occasion. The nurse practitioners felt that because they had to rely on an 'honest' presentation of symptoms, it was inevitable that some patients would be accepted erroneously if this were not forthcoming.

The nurse practitioners were asked what they felt was necessary in order to collect the information needed on which to base a decision at telephone triage. All the nurse practitioners felt that experience and knowledge were the most important factors in making the correct decision within the telephone triage situation. One nurse practitioner felt that it was the nurse practitioner training that had enabled her to gain good questioning skills and to know what information was important. She felt that the experience of interviewing patients face to face at a consultation enabled her to use the same skills on the telephone. Questioning skills were also rated as highly important by other practitioners.

The nurse practitioners felt that the guidelines and criteria for acceptance were of use as a basic pointer (although one nurse practitioner said that she could not remember what the guidelines said and therefore relied totally on her knowledge of whether or not the patient needed to be seen urgently). The two least experienced practitioners tended to consider the guidelines to be of more use to them, whereas those who were more experienced did not use them to any great extent. All the nurse practitioners felt that they might, at times, accept patients who did not fit into the guidelines, because of what was described as a 'gut feeling' about the situation and information surrounding particular patients. This 'gut feeling' was explored further in all the interviews.

One nurse practitioner felt that sometimes:

> it is almost a gut instinct – the history sounds simple, treatable or not urgent but it is utilizing the knowledge that we have to read between the lines, to almost get information from the pauses between the verbal information that you actually get, which is difficult over a telephone and requires an awful lot of clinical experience.

Another felt that the 'gut feeling' was based on knowledge, experience and what had been seen in the past – textbook cases and odd cases of which the practitioner was reminded in a particular situation. Other nurses described 'jumps' from a symptom or odd comment to a knowledge by the nurse practitioner of what was going on in this particular case, and considered that this feeling of definite knowledge and 'gut feeling' was very strong.

The theme of 'gut feeling/reaction' was developed further, and intuition was mentioned. One nurse practitioner said:

> I don't think so – it's what you know – a fast decision about all the facts – do it in your head – it strikes you as being that [a particular diagnosis] before you've got all the symptoms – often with neuro cases: brain tumours and things. It rings a bell even though there are not necessarily classic signs.

Another felt that the phenomenon might be known as intuition but was actually:

> based upon the depth of knowledge you have that you don't even realise you have and the speed at which you use it.

She felt that:

> you don't necessarily think or know why you've got to where you've got to even though you know on paper – everything verbal and what you've got on paper points in a different direction.

One of the other nurse practitioners felt that although intuition might be a valid concept, it could not occur when the patient was not present, and felt that the decisions made were based on asking good questions that satisfied the needs of the nurse practitioner, and that making a fast decision was based on a massive amount of experience – the normal decision-making steps being bypassed.

The general consensus, therefore, was that a vast amount of background knowledge and experience was needed to synthesize the available information very quickly, to read between the lines and to come to an accurate decision with respect to the patient. Protocols were felt to be of little value except as a very rough guide:

> if you just work to protocols you are going to miss things because you don't read the pauses or inferences.

This echoes the study by Elstein and Bordage (1979), who examined doctors' 'intuitive' decision-making and found that a cognitive strategy was in fact used, in which hypotheses were built and further cues directed towards whether to refute or confirm these until a conclusion was reached.

The information elicited from the nurse practitioners at interview clearly echoes Benner's (1984) argument that expert practitioners view situations holistically and draw on past, concrete experience. The nurse practitioners accept the fact of 'gut feeling' or 'intuition', but go on to rationalize this into a collection of experience of similar clinical presentations, expertise, good questioning and expert decision-making rather than the 'nurses know that there is something wrong but cannot explain what it is' type of intuitive feeling suggested by Kenny (1994).

The nurse practitioners seemed able to verbalize the process of decision-making, and in fact often do so in practice in order to confirm, with their peers, their interpretation of a situation. The fact that the less experienced practitioners tended to feel that protocols for acceptance were of more use to them tends to confirm ideas of expert decision-making.

The nurse practitioners also used other factors, such as medical, social and contextual issues, to arrive at a judgement and felt able to interpret non-verbal cues – even during telephone triage – to enable them to arrive at a decision, which echoes the findings of Edwards (1994). Ethical factors also seemed to be taken into account: nurses feeling that patients who were presenting to telephone triage had problems and 'when they need sorting, they shouldn't be messed about'.

One nurse practitioner felt that it might be easier to accept the patient for the Emergency Eye Centre and deal with a trivial problem there rather than send the patient to the GP, who might well after a period of time send the patient to the ARC anyway.

These interviews tend to echo previous authors' ideas of expert decision-making (Benner 1983, Tanner et al 1987, Edwards 1994) and the place of tacit knowledge in practice (Polanyi 1967, Schön 1987). The practitioners have rationalized 'intuition' for themselves into expert knowledge and decision-making, confirming Schön's (1987) ideas of the expert practitioner's skills and reflective processes of 'knowing'.

Limitations of the study

When this study was undertaken, there was a team of very experienced nurse practitioners, a large enough number to staff both departments adequately, who were part of a longstanding team. Because of various changes in role and personnel movement, this is, however, not true at the time of writing up the research study. A high level of questioning skills, decision-making and safety has been demonstrated by the study, but this level may no longer be an accurate reflection of the service. There is less likelihood of an experienced nurse practitioner undertaking telephone triage in either area, and although the member of staff will still be an experienced ophthalmic nurse, the level of experience in the A&E setting may be reduced.

The researcher feels that the literature review may have pointed her in particular directions with regard to ideas of expert decision-making, thus influencing the areas that were examined. This does not detract from the findings, which tend to confirm the results and the ideas of other authors, but may have narrowed the field of inquiry to exclude anything 'new'. There may, of course, be nothing 'new' to find.

A further concern of the researcher is that the nurse practitioners interviewed are part of a close team, of which the researcher is a member. Although the researcher was very careful not to lead or prejudge the nurse practitioners' responses in the interview situation, it is impossible to know how the practitioners influence each other's ideas and how one practitioner's concerns become the concerns of all.

Finally, the small number involved in each of the various categories studied precluded the use of descriptive statistics in this study. A major research study, involving a much higher number of referrals, would be needed in order to investigate statistical significance rather than the trends examined here.

Conclusion

The examination of the results of this research, related to its original aims, shows that the aims have been comprehensively fulfilled. The dynamic research design has enabled the researcher to examine the issues in a greater depth than was first envisaged, leading to a comprehensive view of the workload of both the ARC and the Emergency Eye Centre, the quality of decision-making within the A&E service, and the actual methods by which expert nurse practitioners make these decisions. This study reflects the work undertaken by other authors in other decision-making situations, both when examining telephone triage decisions and in other situations. This study therefore adds to the body of knowledge surrounding expert decision-making.

From the point of view of the practice situation – the A&E service at Manchester Royal Eye Hospital – it is clear that in a high proportion of cases, nurses are able to ascertain an accurate idea of what patients are likely to be presenting to the department, allowing an accurate prediction of the workload. It seems clear that both nurse practitioners and users of the service can be reassured that the decision not to accept patients into the service but to give advice or suggest strategies for more appropriate referral is based on a sound body of knowledge and is safe.

The study should prove to be of use to practitioners, managers and users of the service. Areas of concern were highlighted, which, if pursued, should add to the service. Managers and users of the A&E service have an interest in the financial aspects of the service. Issues such as the possible costs and benefits of a telephone triage system, and of the use of nursing rather than medical staff, provide areas for further research that might concentrate on purely financial perspectives.

It is clear that nurse practitioners have major problems in obtaining a useful history from, in particular, some GPs. This issue needs to be addressed with some urgency, and until it is, neither the hospital not the GP is likely to get the best value from the service. Further education may be required, as well as updates on the success of the service. It might be useful to highlight the expertness of the nurse practitioner, who if presented to the GP as a highly skilled ophthalmic professional, might encounter fewer problems.

References

Atkinson P, Reid M, Sheldrake P (1977) Medical mystique. Sociology of Work and Occupations 4(3): 243–80.

Bailey A, Hallam K, Hurst K (1987) Triage on trial. Nursing Times 83: 65–6.

Benner PE (1983) Uncovering the knowledge embedded in clinical practice. Image: The Journal of Nursing Scholarship 15(2): 36–41.

Benner PE (1984) From Novice to Expert: Excellence and Power in Clinical Nursing Practice. Menlo Park, CA: Addison-Wesley.

Blythin P (1983) 'Would you like to wait over there?' Nursing Mirror (7 Dec): 36–7.

Blythin P (1988) Triage in the UK. Nursing 3(31): 16–20.

Brennan M (1992) Nursing process in telephone advice. Nursing Management 2(5): 62–6.

Brykczynski KA (1989) An interpretive study describing the clinical judgement of nurse practitioners. Scholarly Inquiry for Nursing Practice 3(2): 75–104.

Buckles E, Carew-McColl M (1991) Triage by telephone. Nursing Times 87(6): 26–8.

Cliff KS, Wood TCA (1986) Accident and emergency services – the ambulant patient. Hospital Health Service Review (Mar): 74–7.

Collin F (1985) Theory and Understanding: A Critique of Interpretive Social Science. Oxford: Basil Blackwell.

Corcoran RN, Narayan H (1988) Care evaluation: 'thinking aloud' as a strategy to improve clinical decision making. Heart and Lung: The Journal of Critical Care 15: 56–62.

Crouch R (1992) 'Inappropriate attender' in A&E. Nursing Standard 6(27): 7–9.

de Graafe E (1989) A test of medical problem solving scored by nurses and doctors: the handicap of expertise. Medical Education 23: 381–6.

Dunn JM (1985) Warning: giving telephone advice can be hazardous to your professional health. Nursing (Aug): 40–1.

Eaves K (1987) Why we should care in accident and emergency. Nursing Times (5 Aug): 31–3.

Eddy DM, Clanton CH (1979) The art of diagnosis: solving the clinicopathological exercise. In Dowie J, Elstein A (Eds) Professional Judgement: A Reader in Clinical Decision Making. Cambridge: Cambridge University Press, pp 200–11.

Edwards B (1994) Telephone triage: how experienced nurses reach decisions. Journal of Advanced Nursing 19: 717–24.

Eisner EW (1990) The meaning of alternative paradigms for practice. In Guba EG (Ed.) The Paradigm Dialog. London: Sage, pp 88–102.

Elstein AS, Bordage G (1979) Psychology of reasoning. In Dowie J, Elstein A (Eds) Professional Judgement: A Reader in Clinical Decision Making. Cambridge: Cambridge University Press.

Farrington A (1993) Intuition and expert clinical practice in nursing. British Journal of Nursing 2(4): 228–33.

Firestone WA (1990) Accommodation, toward a paradigm praxis dialectic. In Guba EG (Ed.) The Paradigm Dialog. London: Sage, pp 105–24.

Garthe K (1984) Analysis of distinctions between nursing diagnosis related judgements and disease related nursing judgements. In Kim M et al (Eds) Classification of Nursing Diagnosis: Proceedings of the 5th National Conference. St Louis, MO: CV Mosby.

George JE (1976) Emergency nurse triage beware. Emergency Nurse Legal Bulletin (Winter).

Giddens A (1976) New Rules of Sociological Method: A Positive Critique of Interpretive Sociologies. London: Hutchinson.

Glasper A (1993) Telephone triage: a step forward for nursing practice? British Journal of Nursing 2(2): 34–6.

Glasper A, McGrath K (1993) Telephone triage: extending practice. Nursing Standard 7(15): 34–6.

Goodwin L, Goodwin W (1984) Qualitative vs. quantitative research or qualitative and quantitative research. Nursing Research 33: 378–80.

Green J, Dale J (1990) Health education and the inappropriate use of accident and emergency departments: the views of accident and emergency nurses. Health Education Journal 49(4): 157–61.

Guba EG (Ed.) (1990) The Paradigm Dialog. London: Sage.

Henry SB, Le Breck DB, Holzener WL (1989) The effect of verbalisation of cognitive processes on clinical decision making. Research in Nursing and Health 12(3): 187–93.

Jones CS, McGowan A (1989) Self referral to an accident and emergency department for another opinion. British Medical Journal 298: 859–62.

Jones G (1986) Accident and emergency behind the times. Nursing Times 82(4): 30–3.

Kahneman D, Tvesky A (1973) On the psychology of prediction. Psychological Review 80: 237–51.

Kahneman D, Tvesky A (1990) The simulation heuristic. In Kahneman D, Slavic P, Tvesky A (Eds) Judgement under Uncertainty: Heuristics and Biases. New York: Cambridge University Press, pp 201–8.

Kenny C (1994) Nursing intuition: can it be researched? British Journal of Nursing 3(22): 1191–5.

Kernohan SM, Moir PA, Beatie TF (1992) Telephone calls to a paediatric accident and emergency department. Health Bulletin 50(3): 233–6.

Knowles PJ, Cummins RO (1984) ED medical advice telephone calls: who calls and why? Journal of Emergency Nursing 10(6): 283–6.

Kunkler R, Mitchell A (1994) Advice over the telephone. Nursing Times 90(46): 29–30.

Lawler J (1991) Behind the Screens. London: Churchill Livingstone.

Lincoln YS (1990) The making of a constructivist. In Guba EG (Ed.) The Paradigm Dialog. London: Sage, pp 67–87.

McCormack B (1993) Intuition: concept analysis and application to curriculum development. Journal of Clinical Nursing 2: 11–17.

Mallett J, Woolwich C (1990) Triage in accident and emergency departments. Journal of Advanced Nursing 15: 1443–51.

Marklund B, Bengtsson C (1989) Medical advice by telephone at Swedish health care centres: who calls and what are the problems. Family Practice 6: 42–6.

Marklund B, Bengtsson C, Blomkvist S et al (1990) Evaluation of the telephone advisory activity at Swedish primary health care centres. Family Practitioner 7(3): 184–9.

Meerabeau E (1992) Tacit nursing knowledge: an untapped resource or a methodological headache. Journal of Advanced Nursing 17: 108–12.

Miller WL, Crabtree BF (1994) Clinical research. In Denzin NK, Lincoln YS (Eds) Handbook of Quantitative Research. London: Sage, pp 340–52.

Mills J, Webster AL, Wofsy CB et al (1976) Effectiveness of triage in an urban county hospital. Journal of the American College of Emergency Physicians 5(11): 877–82.

Milner PC, Nicholl JP, Williams BT (1988) Variation in demand for A/E departments in England 1974–1984. Journal of Epidemiology and Community Health 43: 274–8.

Murphie A, Marsden E (1992) A&E departments; value for money? Nursing Standard 7(7): 6–7.

Nuttall M (1986) The chaos controller. Nursing Times (14 May): 66–8.

Orme L, Maggs C (1993) Decision making in clinical practice: how do expert nurses, midwives and health visitors make decisions? Nurse Education Today 13: 270–6.

Phillips DC (1990) Postpositivistic science. In Guba EG (Ed.) The Paradigm Dialog. London: Sage, pp 31–45.

Platt H (1962) Accident and Emergency Services – Report of a Subcommittee of the Standing Medical Advisory Committee of CHSC. London: HMSO.

Polanyi M (1967) The Tacit Dimension. London: Routledge & Kegan Paul.

Rausch T, Rund DA (1981) Nurses' clinical judgements. Nursing Management 12(12): 24–6.

Read S, George S, Williams B, Glasgow J, Potter T (1992) Piloting an evaluation of triage. International Journal of Nursing Studies 29(3): 275–88.

Rock D, Pledge M (1991) Priorities of care for the walking wounded. Triage in accident and emergency. Professional Nurse 6(8): 463–5.

Rund DA, Rausch TS (1981) Triage. St Louis, MO: CV Mosby.

Schön DA (1987) Educating the Reflective Practitioner. San Francisco: Jossey-Bass.

Schön DA (1991) The Reflective Practitioner: How Professionals Think in Action. Avebury: Arena.

Schwant TA (1994) Constructivist, interpretivist approaches to human inquiry. In Denzin NK, Lincoln YS (Eds) Handbook of Qualitative Research. London: Sage, pp 118–37.

Stetson NG (1986) Telephone triage in the ambulatory care setting. Journal of Ophthalmic Nursing and Technology 5(6): 219–22.

Tanner CA, Padrick KP, Westfall UE, Putzier DJ (1987) Diagnostic reasoning strategies of nurses and nursing students. Nursing Research 36(6): 358–63.

Thayre K (1985) Innovations in A&E. Nursing Mirror 60(13): xii–xvi.

Thompson JD, Davies JE (1982) Comprehensive Triage – a Manual for Developing and Implementing a Nursing Care System. Virginia: Reston Publishing.

Timpka T, Arborelius E (1990) The primary care nurse's dilemmas: a study of knowledge use and need during telephone consultations. Journal of Advanced Nursing 15: 1457–65.

Vayer JS, Ten Eyck RP, Cowan ML (1986) New concepts in triage. Annals of Emergency Medicine 15(8): 927–30.

Wheeler SQ (1989) ED Telephone triage: lessons learned from unusual calls. Journal of Emergency Nursing 15(6): 481–7.

Wilkins CV (1992) Paediatric hotline: meeting the needs of the community while conserving health care dollars. Unpublished, Hospital for Sick Kids, Toronto.

Williams DG (1992) Sorting out triage. Nursing Times 88(30): 34–6.

Wood TCA, Cliff KS (1986) Accident and emergency departments – why people attend with minor injuries and ailments. Public Health 100: 15–20.

Worth C, Hurst K (1989) False alarm? Nursing Times 85(15): 24–7.

Yates DW (1987) Nurse triage in the accident and emergency department. Journal of the Royal Society of Health 4: 153–4.

Index

Printed in the United Kingdom
by Lightning Source UK Ltd.
113807UKS00003B/345